KT-583-782

Occupational Therapy
and
Multiple Sclerosis

Occupational Therapy and Multiple Sclerosis

LESLEY SILCOX MPhil, Dip CoT
Occupational Therapist

Illustrations
Colin Smith

Consulting editor in Occupational Therapy
Clephane Hume

MEDICAL LIBRARY
WATFORD POSTGRADUATE
MEDICAL CENTRE
WATFORD GENERAL HOSPITAL
VICARAGE ROAD
WATFORD WD1 8HB

W
WHURR PUBLISHERS
LONDON AND PHILADELPHIA

© 2003 Whurr Publishers

First published 2003 by
Whurr Publishers Ltd
19b Compton Terrace, London N1 2UN, England
325 Chestnut Street, Philadelphia PA19106, USA

Reprinted 2004

All rights reserved. No part of this publication may be
reproduced, stored in a retrieval system, or transmitted
in any form or by any means, electronic, mechanical,
photocopying, recording or otherwise, without the prior
permission of Whurr Publishers Limited.

This publication is sold subject to the conditions that it
shall not, by way of trade or otherwise, be lent, resold,
hired out, or otherwise circulated without the
Publisher's prior consent, in any form of binding or
cover other than that in which it is published, and
without a similar condition including this condition
being imposed upon any subsequent purchaser.

British Library Cataloguing in Publication Data

A catalogue record for this book is available from the
British Library.

ISBN 1 86156 348 5

Contents

Preface

This book is intended for occupational therapists new to the profession who need to know more about multiple sclerosis (MS) and the occupational therapy techniques that can help people with MS. In particular it is aimed at those who work in a general hospital or community setting where they meet only a few people with MS, often when they are most absorbed in their own fears and least able to communicate their needs and abilities. A number of books have been written about MS, from medical texts to personal accounts of living with the disease. There is, however, very little comprehensive information that relates the facts and experience of MS to the management and treatment techniques available to occupational therapists.

The first chapter is a brief description of the history, symptoms, medical treatment and psychological adjustment to MS. Following this, occupational therapy assessment is described including those assessment tools that are currently available. The basic management techniques for the control of physical symptoms, cognitive problems and activities of daily living are described. Work, fatigue, leisure, mobility, the home, issues relating to the later stages of the disease including pressure care and carers are discussed in individual chapters. The final chapter contains contact addresses for MS Societies, equipment suppliers and other useful addresses that are mentioned in the text.

The practical information is the product of the author's 15 years' work as an occupational therapist in Marie Therese House, the rehabilitation unit of the county of Cornwall. Much of the content comes from those people in Cornwall who have MS and are generous in sharing their experience and solutions that have worked for them. Two people in particular have provided long accounts of aspects of their experience of MS that hopefully give a sense of reality to the content. The Cornish population of people with MS have been particularly helpful and tolerant in cooperating with research into occupational therapy and fatigue. Other members of the multidisciplinary team have had a large input to the knowledge base that produced this book, including physiotherapists, nurses and especially doctors, Chris Evans, Jacinta Morgan, David Thornberry and Elizabeth Winterton.

Lesley Silcox
August 2002

Chapter 1
Multiple Sclerosis

What is Multiple Sclerosis?

Multiple sclerosis (MS) is a chronic, progressive demyelinating disease of the central nervous system. Patches or 'plaques' of sclerotic or hardened fibrous tissue can replace the tissue of the myelin sheath at any point within the brain or spinal cord. Myelin is the fatty substance that surrounds the brain and spinal cord and facilitates the conduction of nerve impulses. After trauma and rheumatological disease MS is the next most important cause of severe disability. Among all disabilities at all ages it is the most common one causing people to need help with the basic activities of daily living (Scheinberg, 1994). However, MS does not significantly alter life expectancy, particularly in the early years, although the rate of suicide is increased sevenfold in people with MS (Weinshenker, 1994). Thomas and Daily (1989) found that approximately 85% of newly diagnosed people would be able to lead independent normal lives and only the 'unlucky minority' would become severely handicapped. However Compston et al. (1993) expected 50% of newly diagnosed people to require walking aids within 15 years and only 10% to have no significant disability. MS often starts with an episode of optic neuritis from which the individual usually makes a full recovery. It can be many years before further symptoms are experienced. Studies have shown that between 30% and 70% of people with isolated optic neuritis will develop MS.

MS is a disease of cool climates; the frequency is higher in temperate zones and Western European populations, and lower in tropical and sub-tropical areas. Poser (1994) made a fascinating case for the early origins of MS. He cited epidemiological studies such as

Davenport (1922), which have shown MS to be most common in people of Scandinavian descent. He then traced the spread of the disease as a by-product of Viking expansion and conquest. Norse people became part of the Norman population that invaded Great Britain, while others moved into Eastern Europe. From there they were particularly active in the Crusades, because of the high rates of pay and owing to the presence of Norse chiefs already in the service of the Byzantine Emperor. They also followed the trade routes into Russia and eventually to China, as well as making trading visits to North America. The implication is that their genes are part of the gene pool of the majority of nations in the northern hemisphere.

As yet no one cause of MS has been identified, but it is thought to be a complex combination of genetic and environmental factors. It is possible that spontaneous or environmental factors trigger the onset of the disease. Hutter and Laing (1996) discussed the possibility of one environmental factor, the protective effects of sunlight acting directly upon the central nervous system. This could possibly explain why MS is a disease of temperate climates. For example in Scandinavian countries, where there is a high incidence of MS, there are long periods in winter when daylight is limited.

Who gets Multiple Sclerosis?

The diagnostic criteria for MS give the age of onset as between the ages of 10 and 50. About 5% of cases have their onset below the age of 16, and 2% below the age of 10. The incidence of MS in the USA (Anderson et al., 1992) was estimated to be between 250 and 350 per 100 000. For the United Kingdom, Compston et al. (1993) suggest that in a population of 250 000 the incidence could vary from 250 in the south to 425 in the North East, with between 12 and 20 new cases each year in that population. MS is not evenly distributed between the sexes: approximately 73% of people with MS are women. Possibly because it is a disease of cool climates 95% of people with MS are Caucasian. In the UK, Minden (1994) found that only 29% of people with MS were working, primarily in white-collar jobs.

Diagnosis of Multiple Sclerosis

Making the diagnosis of MS takes a long time because other conditions have to be excluded. The range of time from the first symptoms to the confirmed diagnosis is from 3 to 6 years. The diagnosis of MS has never been easy or uncontroversial. Poser et al. (1983) chaired a committee that produced diagnostic criteria, particularly for research purposes. These were based on one or two 'attacks', supported by clinical or laboratory evidence. They defined an 'attack' as 'the occurrence of a symptom or symptoms of neurological dysfunction which lasts for more than twenty four hours'. This includes symptoms related to eye movement, coordination, balance, sensation, speech, reflexes and weakness, which are assessed clinically and other possible causes eliminated. Compston et al. (1993) mentioned the use of computed tomography (CT) scanning, magnetic resonance imaging (MRI) and lumbar puncture to aid diagnosis. A lumbar puncture allows the physician to infer that immunological reactions are taking place. Immunoglobulins are antibodies that are made in response to antigens; these are a mixture of certain types of virus that are thought to have a role in triggering MS. The presence of these in the cerebral spinal fluid is evidence that antibodies are being made in the central nervous system.

The use of MRI has recently become the most frequent aid to diagnosis and neurological investigation. The images produced by an MRI scan show 90% of plaques of demyelination in the area scanned. MRI is used to detect active lesions and to measure total lesion load. One of its functions is to improve the understanding of the correlation between clinical events and pathological changes in the nervous system. Poser (1994) expressed some need for caution in its use for diagnosis; he described the proliferation of MRI machines as having already led to a frightening increase in the misdiagnosis of MS.

Imparting the diagnosis to the person affected has been a subject for concern and until recently doctors were reluctant to tell people the diagnosis once it was confirmed. This began to change about 20 years ago. Elian (1985) elicited opinions from a sample of 167 patients with MS. She found that 139 said it was only right to tell the patient straightforwardly the true diagnosis, 22 did not feel strongly either way and only six felt that it should have been kept from them. All felt that the person to impart the information should be the medical consultant. She concluded her investigation by citing the doctor's fear of whether the patient can stand being told. In the light of her findings Elian (1985) asked, 'can the patient stand not being told?' Burnfield (1989a) stated that most people with MS speak with relief at knowing their diagnosis. Naturally many are shocked and distressed, but at least they know the truth and are able to begin to come to terms with it. He concluded that the truth is rarely worse than the unknown, and that honesty could enhance the doctor – patient relationship so leading to greater trust. Compston et al. (1993) gave guidelines for imparting the diagnosis, including the importance of offering sufficient information about the disease, in order that people can begin to plan their own lives.

In the UK, a neurologist who makes the diagnosis may retain care of the individual, or refer him/her to a rehabilitation specialist. This will depend on the procedures in place in each health care trust and should be explained to the individual. Many health districts provide a specialist team of professionals who are able to support the individual and the family once the consultant has explained the diagnosis. These teams develop close relationships with their local branches of the MS Society. There are national branches of the MS Society in most countries where the disease is prevalent. These provide a range of services that vary with the health provision of their respective countries. Services can include treatment, respite care, the provision of equipment, group meetings, information and support to people with MS, their carers and professionals. These societies are coordinated by the International MS Society, which has an excellent website; its address and those of some national branches can be found in Chapter 11.

Forms that Multiple Sclerosis can Take

In some health districts in the UK the medical care available to people with MS may be dependent on the type of MS that they have and the stage that it has reached. It is therefore important to know the terms used for the different forms or stages of the disease. Compston et al. (1993) state that in 80% of cases, MS begins with episodic neurological symptoms, from which people recover fully at first. After this there are a number of patterns which the progress of the disease can take:

(1) *Relapsing–remitting disease*, where people report clearly defined relapses in their disease with full recovery. There is no progression between relapses. A relapse can be a devastating experience, sometimes as severe as general paralysis of the voluntary muscles, bowel and bladder problems and loss of vision. A relapse can necessitate an admission to acute medical care in hospital. A relapse can last from 1 to 6 weeks.

(2) *Primary progressive disease*, which most commonly affects the spinal

cord and is the usual mode of presentation in people in or after the fifth decade.

(3) *Secondary progressive disease*, which tends to affect whichever system has borne the brunt of the earlier disease course. The cerebellar area is more frequently affected than in primary progressive disease. Kidd et al. (1995) suggested that 66% of people with relapsing–remitting disease would subsequently develop secondary progressive disease.

(4) *Benign disease*, which is most common in young females with mainly sensory symptoms who recover completely from individual episodes.

(5) *Malignant disease* can also occur; this form of the disease affects only a small percentage of people but can be fatal. It can result in respiratory failure when the medulla is affected, or massive cerebral demyelination.

(6) *Progressive–relapsing disease* was defined by Lubin and Reingold (1996) as progressive from onset, with clear relapses with or without recovery.

Symptoms of Multiple Sclerosis

Disorders of Movement

Disorders of movement include ataxia, spasticity and muscle weakness, all of which are deviations from normal human movement (Bobath, 1985). One of the main functions of normal movement patterns is economy, ensuring that the body uses the minimum necessary energy for daily activity. Deviance could therefore contribute to the individual's level of fatigue. Ataxia is caused by cerebellar degeneration that results in poor neuromuscular coordination, which manifests itself in shaking or tremor of the limbs, trunk and head. It is one of the most difficult symptoms to treat and is most disabling in the upper limb. Medications have only a damping down effect on the tremor and are likely to produce unacceptable side effects or result in the development of tolerance. Compston et al. (1993) described how the tremors could be modified by relaxing the muscles with comfortable supportive seating and also by avoiding excitement and anxiety. Roberts (1997) added to this list compensatory equipment to facilitate economy of movement and conserve energy.

Spasticity is a common and very disabling symptom that occurs in about 80% of people with MS. It takes the form of hypertonicity of the muscles, impairs walking and causes shortening of soft tissue, which contributes to nursing problems in the more disabled people (Francis, 1993). It is most common in the lower limbs, is worse at night and much worse if the person becomes overheated or has an infection. A specific example of the effects of abnormal muscle tone is clonus, the spasmodic alteration of muscle contraction and relaxation at a regular frequency, induced by stretch. This is most common in the legs and is seen in regular tapping of the heel where weight is placed through the ball of the foot rather than the heel. There are several drugs available to manage increased tone, which need to be carefully adjusted for the individual and reassessed regularly. These include:

- *baclofen*: acts on neurotransmitters, decreasing the firing of the motor neuron, but may produce muscle weakness and drowsiness;
- *dantrolene*: acts peripherally but is only used if other drugs are not effective because it can produce serious side effects including liver damage;
- *diazepam*: enhances the action of inhibitory neurotransmitters; it is less effective for the relief of spasticity but helps to relieve anxiety and aids relaxed sleep;
- *tizanadine*: acts on the synaptic spinal excitatory pathways, does not produce muscle weakness but can have a sedative effect;
- *cannabis*: is arousing much public and political interest; it has been shown to be effective, although it is not yet known whether this effect is better than any other preparation;
- *intrathecal baclofen*: can be used with an indwelling pump, which supplies precise doses of the drug at exact intervals (Porter, 1997). The dose and frequency can be programmed remotely, without physical intrusion. The pump is effective but requires careful monitoring, refilling with baclofen and a surgical procedure to replace it after approximately 5 years when the batteries wear out.
- *botulinum*: toxin type A(BT/A) is also given by injection to treat spasticity in specific target muscles; this is effective but requires to be repeated every 3 to 6 months (Wantanbe et al., 1998).

The treatment of spasticity, however, also requires some self-help, physiotherapy and occupational therapy advice. This may include amended positions for sitting and lying in bed, exercise, stretching either alone or with a helper and changes in the daily routine.

Muscle weakness of the extremities is a frequent symptom of MS, usually due to reduced action of the motor nervous system on the muscles. Muscles that are not stimulated by their nerves and therefore not used soon become wasted, unless specific exercises are performed regularly. Exercise is particularly important when recovering from a relapse. There is currently no medical treatment available to help muscle weakness. Roberts (1997) advised physiotherapy and occupational therapy intervention, but rehabilitation from this weakness is made more difficult because neuromuscular fatigue hampers muscle strengthening

Fatigue

Fatigue has been defined (Krupp and Pollina, 1996) as 'an overwhelming sense of tiredness, lack of energy, and feeling of exhaustion. It is different from the symptoms of depression, which include lack of self-esteem, despair or feelings of hopelessness; it is also distinguished from limb weakness.' Freal et al. (1984) conducted one of the first studies of fatigue in MS. Their sample group consisted of 656 patients, of whom 78% were found to suffer from fatigue, and 56% of the group found their fatigue so severe as to cause them to have problems with activities of daily living. The symptoms of fatigue that their respondents described included 'weakness', 'tiredness', 'need to rest', 'heat makes it worse' and 'other symptoms more apparent'. Fatigue was seen to be always present but at its most disabling in the late afternoon; two-thirds of the sample experienced it daily or almost daily. In 47% the fatigue subsided within a few hours, and 40% reported varying durations for their periods of fatigue. Freal et al. (1984) stated that given the known pathology of MS the fatigue reported by people with MS is probably not due to muscular pathology. Neither was it likely to be a psychosomatic phenomenon, given the high proportion of the MS population with fatigue symptoms. Kielhofner (1985) discussed occupational therapy in MS fatigue only one year after the results of this initial study of fatigue were published. This possibly indicates that occupational therapists have long considered fatigue to be a symptom of MS that they could treat effectively.

Krupp et al. (1989) found that 28% of a sample of people with MS described their fatigue as 'the worst symptom'. Fatigue, according to Burnfield (1989c) may be experienced as overwhelming tiredness or as sensory difficulties, including blurred vision, slurred speech, pins and needles and numbness. It can be brought on by exertion, heat, infection, or overeating. When experienced, the signs and symptoms of MS are more pronounced. He suggested that the fatigue felt by people with MS was rather different from that experienced by the general population, because the nervous system was involved as well as the muscles. The medical treatment for fatigue has been amantadine or pemoline, both of which have been researched and found to be only moderately effective. Most recently modafinil, a drug approved for narcolepsy, has been found to be more effective without being addictive or producing the severe side effects.

Problems of Continence

Impaired control of bowel or bladder affects about 33% of people with MS. Bladder function can be affected by demyelination in the medial frontal lobes, the pons or the spinal cord, giving rise to irritative symptoms that cause storage problems and difficulty in initiating voiding. Irritative symptoms and incomplete emptying may coexist and cause the presence of residual urine that may exacerbate frequency, urgency and the risk of infection. Time and careful, tactful questioning may be required when discussing this with people. Thompson (1996) described the management of continence as one of the areas of greatest medical improvement in recent years including drug regimens, and more effective methods of catheterization and intermittent self-catheterization. Pelvic floor exercises are also recommended.

Bowel problems for people with MS are more likely to be manifested in constipation than faecal incontinence. Compston et al. (1993) found 10% of known people with MS to have problems of constipation and only 4% incontinence. This is because the normal gastric reflexes and peristaltic contractions are affected by demyelination. Decreased sensation and spasticity in the rectum and anus results in delayed defecation and therefore moisture is absorbed back into the system. The person's reduced mobility means that the intestinal contents are not stimulated to move quickly. Constipation can also result from some forms of medication. Methods of regulating the emptying of the bowel include the carefully monitored use of aperients, suppositories and enemas. Also, bulking agents and increased fibre in the diet are encouraged and again the teaching and use of pelvic floor exercises.

Dizziness, Unsteadiness and Disturbance of Proprioception

Dizziness in MS can be due to visual impairment and must be distinguished from dizziness due to postural hypotension. The symptoms are commonly due to impaired vestibular mechanisms, and tend to fluctuate and to remit spontaneously. Schapiro et al. (1997) explained that mild non-specific dizziness or giddiness occurred as an initial symptom in 5% to 9% of patients with MS and that attacks of true vertigo do occur, either initially or as part of a relapse. Compston et al. (1993) suggested that some people describe their problem as dizziness when they experience clumsy movements in limbs and trunk or, because of reduced sensation, are not aware of the position of their limbs in space. Disturbed proprioception, the loss of the sensation of movement and the position of the limbs, causes uncertainty and clumsiness of movement. In MS, this tends to have its most severe effect on the legs, and is only countered by prolonged physiotherapy.

Visual Disturbance

Visual disturbances are a familiar symptom of MS, because the optic nerve is particularly susceptible to demyelination, being structurally part of the brain rather than a true nerve. Inflammation of the optic nerve can also cause diplopia (double vision), transient visual loss, or blurring of vision. Schapiro and Langer (1994) noted that almost all people with MS have or will have visual symptoms. Visual problems that occur as part of a relapse can be treated by the use of steroids and low vision aids. Pre-existing visual problems may be accentuated by demyelination of the optic nerve and it is therefore important that people who already wear spectacles should have their eyes checked regularly. In some cases a unilateral frosted lens in spectacles or an eye patch may be used for diplopia. Franklin and Burks (1985) found that nystagmus also occurs, sometimes severe enough to affect reading.

Loss of Sensation and Pain

Sensory problems that occur in MS result from the loss of myelin from the sensory nerves, including reduced tactile sensation. The individual may feel as if there was a film of cloth over the skin, band-like dysesthesia round the chest, which makes breathing feel difficult, or, less commonly, a band around the abdomen. Coldness, pins and needles, tingling, heat or tight, swollen sensations of the extremities are often reported and facial changes, which may be similar to trigeminal neuralgia, may occur.

Pain in MS also can be due to damage to the nervous system that results in inappropriate or confused messages reaching the brain. Although it has been recognized as a symptom of MS from the earliest documentation, the idea that it is uncommon seems to remain. The evidence shows some form of pain to be present in 64% of people with MS, and for 10% the pain is acute (Thompson, 1996). It increases with age, is more intense in females than males, can have an effect on mental health and has a substantial effect on social role (Archibald et al., 1994). It also has a considerable effect on quality of life (Gilmore and Strong, 1998). Spasm is a common cause of the pain reported by people with MS, resulting from muscular stiffness, actual involuntary muscle action and the conscious attempt to control it. The treatment for pain is mainly pharmacological and should be covered in the comprehensive care package. However, because pain does not correlate with disease characteristics, it needs to be evaluated on an individual basis. Other remedies include transcutaneous nerve stimulation (TNS), and some of the less conventional approaches such as biofeedback, acupuncture, meditation, visualization and yoga. Finally, and as suggested by people with MS, it may be important for them to examine their attitudes to pain and maintain a positive outgoing attitude to life.

Communication and Swallowing Difficulty

Communication problems can include loss of volume of speech and slurring of speech, both of which may vary during the course of the day, usually deteriorating towards the end of the day. There are several schools of thought about the causes of communication problems among people with MS. Lechtenberg (1988) explained that in speech disorders the fundamental disturbance is in coordinating the movements of the tongue, lips, palate, vocal cords and other elements vital to speech. Alternatively Kujala et al. (1996) attributed these problems to mild cognitive deterioration. Roberts (1997) described the importance of referral to a speech therapist and the possible provision of communication aids. Dysphagia, or difficulty in masticating and swallowing, was considered by Thompson (1996) to be another symptom that seemed to be underestimated. He described it as difficult to treat because it fluctuated with the patient's level of fatigue. Roberts (1997) stated that swallowing cannot be assessed separately from feeding and seating positions, and that a speech and language therapist should be involved. In cases where feeding is lengthy or where there is danger of chest infection from aspiration, a percutaneous endoscopic gastrostomy (PEG) may be recommended.

Problems of Cognition

Cognitive problems in MS have only been recognized comparatively recently. Staples and Lincoln (1979) were out of step with contemporary thinking in the disability movement when they published their paper on intellectual impairment in MS and its impact on functional abilities. Major conclusions of this work were that there was a high frequency of memory impairment, which should be routinely tested. They also concluded that reports of daily living skills given by individual patients could be unreliable and needed to be checked. Burnfield (1989b) discussed problems in the past when these symptoms were either not recognized or over-stressed. He suggested that both people with MS and their partners ended up feeling guilty, misunderstood and isolated. Once they realized that these symptoms had an organic cause, they were in a better position to start to cope with them.

Compston et al. (1993) found that 30% of people with MS had problems with memory overall and 20% had problems of intellectual impairment. Amongst the latter, 10% suffered from mild physical disability and 30% from severe physical disability. Frontal lobe functions such as judgement, decision making and appropriate social behaviour are affected in about 15% of people with MS, again most frequently in those with severe physical disability. All of these problems should be discussed with the patient and the relatives, because the behaviour that results can be misinterpreted by the family or carers as being uncaring or selfish. For individual people with MS, cognitive impairment may be more disruptive to the activities of daily living than the physical symptoms, and may occur early when physical symptoms are minimal. If cognitive impairment is severe it usually accompanies chronic progressive disease, other symptoms of which are ataxia and gait disorder (Mendez, 1995).

Grigsby et al. (1994), in a study of working memory impairment in people with MS, found that there were limitations on the amount of information that could be processed and retained. This would make it difficult to solve complex tasks efficiently; people with MS must rely on more deliberate, conscious control of their activity. With progressive disease, this control is liable to become increasingly inefficient and more errors will occur. This may explain why patients complain that they are unable to keep track of two tasks at the same time, or to remember their intended actions. This finding has implications for treatment programmes that require the individual to take control of his/her own activities. Problems in decision making and judgement may make it difficult for people to participate in a treatment programme that requires the skills of planning and goal setting.

Disorders of Mood

Emotional responses to MS include depression, grieving, a sense of loss, and a feeling of distress for both the individual and the family. Two other emotional states more specifically associated with MS are chronic sorrow and euphoria. The most common of these responses is depression, with a direct relationship between severity of disability and severity of depression. Sadovnick et al. (1996) studied the relationship between depression and MS and suggested that depression was understandable in chronic debilitating illness. However, the rate of depression in MS was consistently higher than in other chronic debilitating illnesses. They found that 53% of their sample of people with MS had symptoms of depression by the end of their fifth decade. These symptoms are described by Jablow (1998, p. 3) as:

- feelings of hopelessness, sadness and despair;
- loss of pleasure or interest in most activities;
- significant weight loss or gain; or increase or decrease in appetite;
- persistent sleep problems, either insomnia or excessive sleep;
- ongoing fatigue and loss of energy;
- feeling of personal worthlessness or inappropriate guilt;
- observable restlessness or slowed movement;
- recurrent thoughts of death, violence or suicide.

The person with MS has to deal with the uncertainties of his or her situation, which is virtually a life sentence. This evokes an emotional state that has been described as chronic sorrow. Hainsworth (1994) defined chronic sorrow as a pervasive sadness that is permanent, periodic and progressive, an emotional pain that may lie dormant but be activated by reminders of unfulfilled life goals. Because MS is a chronic condition and for some people may be life threatening, the sorrow that people feel because of it may also become chronic. Chronic sorrow also affects relatives of people with MS, especially spouses; it is often present when lifestyle is disrupted and every experience of discomfort increases the fear of developing debilitating MS. Mourning cannot alleviate this situation.

Euphoria is an altered mood state that is often associated with MS; it is defined as sustained elevation of mood or inappropriate sense of well-being. Roberts (1997) confirmed that euphoria has been given undue prominence in MS; it is probably present in under 10% of people.

Sexual Problems

Sexuality is a far more complex aspect of human interaction than just a physical sexual relationship. It includes the whole of a person's interaction with other people, expressions of an individual's need to be attractive, self-esteem and perception of body image. It is also involved with the ability to fulfil appropriate social and cultural roles. These aspects are less recognized than the known medical ones that Thompson (1996) described as common in MS, and are probably still under-recognized by health professionals.

The sexual symptoms that were most difficult for people with MS are described by Valleroy and Kraft (1984). For women the major problem was fatigue, followed by decreased sensation and libido. For men the main problems were achieving and maintaining an erection, decreased sensation and fatigue. Frequent urinary tract infections were cited as a severe problem by a smaller number of people. Loss of sexual potency has been found to be associated with neurogenic bladder dysfunction and pyramidal impairment of the lower limbs. Sexual libido can also be reduced by symptoms of MS including pain, spasticity and sensory changes, or as a side effect of some medications.

Erectile failure can be successfully managed by sildenafil (Viagra), papaverine injections and, as reported by Heller et al. (1992), by vacuum tumescence constriction. Schapiro (Schapiro and Langer, 1994) mentioned other options such as vibration, vaginal lubricating packets and alternative methods of expressing sexuality. Most of the literature on the physical expression of sexuality (Rabin, 1980; Siosteen et al., 1990) has been written by or for people who have spinal injuries but most of this advice is applicable to people with MS. Rabin (1980) provides illustrations of the most effective positions to achieve sexual contentment and satisfaction.

Medical Treatment of Multiple Sclerosis

The working party of the British Society of Rehabilitation Medicine (Compston et al., 1993) confirmed that there is at present no drug or dietary treatment that can cure or prevent the onset of MS. Drug therapy is currently used in three ways: first, steroids are used to reduce oedema around the inflammatory MS lesion, because there will be no remyelination while oedema is present (Hommes, 1997).

Steroids do not affect the disease process, only the immediate symptoms of relapse. They are given in hospital in high doses and occasionally the person reacts to the treatment with a form of mania, the mildest form of which is garrulousness. Second, use of medication attempts to restore nerve conductivity in demyelinated nerve fibres, by prolongation of the repolarization phase of the action potential (Smits et al., 1994). Third, drugs can alter the immune balance of the body, in the hope that the process of demyelination will be slowed down (McDonald, 1995). Roberts (1997) mentioned intravenous methylprednisolone, which has been shown to decrease the duration of relapse but not to influence the outcome.

Currently, the interferon group of drugs is being developed for the treatment of MS. With the advent of interferon beta, Ebers (1994) described the mood among colleagues as 'now approaching optimism'. Research is moving quickly. Liblau and Fontaine (1998) reviewed recent advances and experimental evidence on the action of interferon beta in MS and found new therapeutic possibilities and a better understanding of its immunopathology. These drugs, alone or in combination, provide hope for better treatment for at least some subgroups of people with MS. In the UK there remains a reluctance to use these drugs mainly on grounds of cost, but also due to the need for further research. When prescribed they are usually considered appropriate only for people with relapsing–remitting disease. The National MS Society is attempting to get this decision reversed. Continuing positive research evidence may help their case.

Although it is not at present possible to cure or prevent MS, it is possible to assist people through the treatment of symptoms. Scheinberg (1994) told his audience that the advances in the management of the disease have been achieved as a result of directing attention to specific symptoms in MS patients and not to any scientific advances that have been made. He made a strong case for the consultant neurologist to play a very active role in informing and educating the patient. He concluded: 'Most of what we do in the improvement of our MS patients is through the patient's own abilities, by exposure to rehabilitative measures'.

Measurement of Disability

Disability in MS was first measured by Kurtzke using the Disability Status Scale (Kurtzke, 1955); this is an 11-point ordinal scale from 0 (normal) to 10 (death from MS). He has continued to work in this field and among other works (Kurtzke, 1983) published the Expanded Disability Status Scale (EDSS), which introduced halfway stages between the 11 points of the Disability Status Scale, making a 20-point scale (0 and 10 remain unchangeable). The EDSS is used as the standard measure in virtually all research related to MS. It is often used in conjunction with Kurtzke's Functional Systems (Kurtzke, 1955), which scores the functions of eight systems: the pyramidal, cerebellum, brainstem, sensory, bowel and bladder, visual, cerebral, and 'other' – which includes spasticity.

A standard measure of disability for MS, the Minimal Record of Disability (Haber and LaRocca, 1985), which includes Kurtzke's scales, has been designed and tested in conjunction with the International Federation of MS Societies. Its intention is to improve communication on the care of people with MS. It is expected that the information generated by the scale will be useful in planning for people with other chronic neurological conditions, and to provide valuable information to planners of health services and health economists. This is now the standard measure in the USA, it is short and simple to complete and has its own instruction booklet. There is no evidence that it has yet reached regional rehabilitation services within the UK. It is a team document requiring the input of several health care disciplines to complete.

Diet and Multiple Sclerosis

Diet is an important topic among people with MS. A great many diets have been designed and published but there is little evidence of the effectiveness of most of these. Some individuals place great faith in them and to shatter that faith could have a negative effect on the person concerned. The MS Society (Reeves, 1995) does not recommend either the allergy diet or the gluten-free diet. It does, however, recommend a healthy diet containing all five groups of nutrients. The number of calories that an individual needs will depend upon his/her level of activity, and will decline if he/she becomes less active with progressive disease. There is therefore a danger of weight gain as the person becomes less active; should this happen the individual is advised to reduce his/her intake of sugar and fats. Other dietary advice includes the importance of fibre to maintain bowel health, and vitamins for skin nutrition and to help with the metabolism of iron and calcium, as reduced levels of both of these can be problems for people with MS. Alcohol is considered safe in moderation, but someone with MS may experience its effects more quickly.

On a more positive note the MS Society (Reeves, 1995) recommends the use of polyunsaturated fats because they have been shown to have some relationship to the reduction of the severity and duration of relapses. This is because polyunsaturated fatty acids are important to the maintenance of nerve fibres. They are components of cell membranes and the myelin sheath, which is damaged in MS, is a cell membrane. Polyunsaturated fatty acids are also involved in making prostaglandins, which are involved in the immune system.

Acceptance of Multiple Sclerosis

The way in which an individual and his or her close relatives come to terms with the diagnosis of MS is very important to everybody who comes into contact with them. Knowledge of the process of acceptance will help the professional to understand some of the behaviour that they may encounter. Occupational therapists may be aware of the use of a 'bereavement model' of coping with loss to describe coming to terms with disability. This describes the progress through anger and then denial to acceptance. For MS a more complex model has been in use for many years. It was discussed by Evers and Karnilowicz (1996), who conducted a large sample study of the psychosocial ramifications of MS and people's ability to handle social and emotional life. Their conclusion was that people were not homogeneous in their psychosocial characteristics and that factors other than duration of disease were important. They suggested that the current literature presents an unnecessarily bleak picture to newly diagnosed people, especially when it is remembered that only a minority of people diagnosed with MS will become severely disabled. In their study frequent references were made to a classic paper on adjustment to MS by Matson and Brooks (1977).

'Adjusting to multiple sclerosis' was an exploratory study by Matson and Brooks (1977), who discussed psychosocial adjustment to MS. The paper stressed the importance of 'improvement in self-concept, mediated by the degree of impairment associated with the disease process'. There was no simple, linear relationship between increased duration of disease and better self-concept. Matson and Brooks (1977, p. 249) defined four stages in adjustment to MS:

- *Denial*: 'It can't be true: it can't be happening to me'. Concealing symptoms. Seeking an authority who will deny the diagnosis. Refusing help. Holding to past life and values.

- *Resistance*: 'It won't get me down'. Searching for a cure or treatment. Active in programmes: seeking other patients. Reluctance to accept help. Initial recognition of change in life orientation.
- *Affirmation*: 'I guess I have to face it'. Grieving for loss of former self. Publicly explaining about MS. Learning to accept help. Subjectively rearranging priorities in life.
- *Integration*: 'I know it's there, but I don't think much about it'. Living with it. Spending time and energy on other matters. Accepting help when necessary. Integration of lifestyle with new values.

It is often not until the third, affirmation stage that people are able to accept help, and to rearrange their priorities in life. At the first denial stage people may not hear what is being said to them, even if they are prepared to listen. It is important to have a member of the family or friend with them so that the information that is given is not lost. They may be angry or dismissive, making it very difficult to form any sort of professional relationship with them. Some elements of the resistance stage may be positive: people look for cures and try everything from diets to yoga to hyperbaric oxygen. Sometimes they actually find an activity that does help, if only in assisting them to relax or by channelling their energy in new directions. Alternatively there are a number of people who have been known to move from a level home environment to a house, in order to use the stairs for exercise. The understanding of these attitudes can help health care professionals to accept the individual's needs and to wait, however reluctantly, to be asked to help. Walsh and Walsh (1987) added to this model with their study of self-esteem in people with MS. They found that self-esteem varied with the stage of adaptation. Further to this, Wassem (1992) stated that adjustment occurs when the disability no longer uses up all the individual's energy and so energy is freed for other activities.

This understanding of personal adjustment to MS is described by Handron (1993), herself a health care professional with MS. She explained the use of denial to maintain the delicate balance between vulnerability and strength. The struggle to gain a new vision of reality after the diagnosis of a serious illness is a long-term process. She insisted that clinical interventions directly confronting the denial mechanism are ineffective and non-therapeutic, and can even increase the person's anxiety and need for denial. She wrote:

> On a good day denial may serve to bolster and support a person in
> getting on with a life that is worth living. On bad days denial may
> provide the rationale for an impulsive action or poor decision.
> (Handron, 1993, p. 29)

As a conclusion to this chapter the following excerpt is taken from an
interview with a lady who has MS. She is now in her early seventies,
moderately disabled but organizing the care for her elderly husband.
This quotation puts the realities described by Matson and Brooks
(1977) into everyday language.

> I did not want anybody to know, when I first had it I did not want
> anybody to know there was something wrong with me and I did a sort
> of vanishing act. I did not want to go out and got depressed and every-
> thing, a real clinical depression, I did not want to see anybody with MS
> or to know about the MS society or anything. So eventually ... I thought
> everybody was wrong and that everybody was awful to me, it was not so
> at all, it was just me enlarging on everything. And the social services
> would come here and they would depress me because they would
> suggest things ... like 'have you thought of sort of trying a wheelchair?'
> That was when I could not balance or anything and that depressed me.
> Anyway eventually I had some tablets for the depression after nine
> months and it made a world of difference. Then someone rang and
> said, 'Why don't you join the MS Society?' and they were from the MS
> Society, Oh I know who it was, she used to be almoner, she was our
> social worker for the MS Society. She said, 'Why don't you join the MS
> Society?' and I said oh no, but I would not mind being put in touch with
> somebody like myself, with it to the same degree as me with a family like
> me and roughly on the same scale, so she did. From then on I talked
> and talked to Margaret who had also done the same thing and she had
> found her way and I found my way. From then on I was ... I consider
> myself OK.

Summary

(1) MS is a chronic progressive demyelinating disease of the central
     nervous system that does not significantly affect life expectancy.
     Only a minority of people with MS will become severely
     disabled.
(2) Between 250 and 350 in each 100 000 of the population have
     MS; 73% of them are women and 95% are Caucasian.
(3) The diagnosis of MS is made based on one or two 'attacks' with
     symptoms of neurological dysfunction. Recently, magnetic
     resonance imaging has been used to aid the diagnosis.

(4) The forms that MS can take are: relapsing–remitting disease, primary progressive disease, secondary progressive disease, benign disease, malignant disease, and progressive–relapsing disease.

(5) The symptoms of MS are disorders of movement, fatigue, problems with continence, dizziness, unsteadiness and disturbance of proprioception, visual disturbance, loss of sensation and pain, difficulty in communication and swallowing, problems of cognition, disorders of mood, and sexual problems.

(6) There is at present no drug or other treatment that can cure or prevent the onset of MS, although with interferon beta there is improvement in relapse rate and duration and hope for future research.

(7) The accepted measurement of disability in MS is based on the work of Kurtzke, from the Disability Status Scale (1955) to the Minimal Record of Disability (1985).

(8) Diet in MS is the subject of much discussion; the MS Society does not recommend either the gluten-free diet or the allergy diet. It does, however, recommend a healthy balanced diet and the use of polyunsaturated fats.

(9) A model of the process of coming to accept MS, and a personal account of this, is described.

Chapter 2
Assessment

The assessment process involves occupational therapists in learning about an individual patient, whilst maintaining an awareness of the theory and purpose of the assessment. It is not the intention of this book to discuss the basic theory and practice of the assessment process (Trombly, 1995; Foster, 1996) but to suggest how that theory can be used specifically for the treatment of people with MS. Neither will it attempt to promote a specific model of practice for work with people who have MS; any of the relevant models will provide a theoretical basis for intervention. Those who use model-specific assessment tools will need to consider the relevance to their model of the tools described in the second section of this chapter.

The process of assessment covers all of the occupational therapist's interaction with the patient, from receiving a referral to the point where the individual's data have been collected, analysed and a set of treatment goals defined in discussion with the patient. It may include more than one interview and may involve the use of standardized measurement tools. The data generated during the assessment are objectively analysed using the therapist's knowledge base of the disease, understanding of the measurement tools and the available resources, without any judgemental attitudes, and must include the particular needs of the person's environment and culture.

The Task of Assessment

The assessment of someone with MS can cover a wide spectrum of aspects of the disease including physical, cognitive and emotional areas and environmental constraints. It is usually led by a presenting problem that has precipitated the referral, but should not preclude other areas of investigation if the patient so wishes. It is unfortunately true that for a large proportion of occupational therapists intervention is confined to one assessment followed by problem solving, often involving the provision of equipment or referral to another agency. This approach is not always appropriate for people with MS who, if they will accept it, benefit from ongoing support and intervention (Ashburn and De Souza, 1988).

The Person to be Assessed

At the beginning of the twenty-first century the occupational therapist should be confident that the person referred to her/him does in fact have MS and that this information has been provided by a consultant neurologist. The individual may attend for an appointment with a member of his/her family or a friend, or the therapist may be invited to his/her home. He/she may be newly diagnosed or have lived with the disease for years and had few problems to date. As described in Chapter 1, a newly diagnosed person may be angry or in denial, and her/his companion may have his/her own emotional reaction to the situation. One fact is certain: each person will be individual and different from everybody else with MS. They may all have similar levels of disability and virtually identical problems but they will come from different environments and have diverse coping strategies. Their companions will also have needs, for information, for support, for understanding or just for the whole thing to be taken away. One lady with MS described her husband's response to her diagnosis as, 'he said he felt that he had already lost me'.

It will be important to confirm during the first assessment that the person is aware of and, if appropriate, is receiving all of the available welfare rights benefits. This may not be the role of the occupational therapist in all health care settings, but it is important that the individual receives this information as soon after diagnosis as possible. In the UK the most comprehensive details of benefits can be found in the *Disability Rights Handbook*, details of which are with other sources of information in Chapter 11.

Assessment Location

The context in which the assessment takes place is important to the nature of the therapeutic relationship that can be created with each individual. The individual's own home, an occupational therapy department or a hospital ward all affect that potential relationship in different ways. In a person's home the occupational therapist is a guest, usually invited to the part of the house where visitors are entertained. At home the patient will usually feel more comfortable and in control of the interview. It may be easier there for individuals to explain the problems that they are experiencing with their environment, but they may be more confident in avoiding the discussion of intimate personal matters.

The occupational therapy department is the familiar environment to the therapist and efforts will have to be made to make the atmosphere friendly and relaxed before people being assessed will feel as confident as they do in their own homes. A great deal may be achieved in this area by peer support if a group or small class is available, so that there are people with similar problems who can reassure the new person before therapeutic intervention begins. The hospital ward may be part of the therapist's workplace but patients view it as a medical and nursing area. People will often be much less inhibited about practising personal activities of daily living and discussing intimate problems in a ward situation. To illustrate these differences an occupational therapist described her conversation with Jayne who has MS. Jayne complained bitterly that she had been embarrassed and felt degraded when she was asked by a visiting domiciliary occupational therapist to demonstrate the difficulties that she had with dressing. She had in fact complained to Social Services about this imposition. However, this conversation took place while the occupational therapist was assessing and facilitating her in taking a bath. A hospital-based occupational therapist was acceptable for personal activities of daily living, while another in Jayne's own home was not.

Introducing Occupational Therapy

The first occupational therapist to meet a person with MS has a responsibility to inform that person's understanding about the profession. Those who are to be among the unlucky minority who go on to be severely disabled will be helped by ongoing contact with health care professionals. The first meeting remains in people's memories and failing memory can distort what is recalled. A clear but brief description needs to be given, including what occupational therapy is and what the service can actually offer. Do not be afraid to repeat this, rephrased if possible, because people tend not to take in everything that is explained to them. Consider basing a description of the role of occupational therapy on the following quotation from Kielhofner (1992, p. 243), relating to the difference between the occupational therapy approach and other professions:

> ... the therapeutic approach does not stress interventions aimed at primarily altering the course and consequence of the disease. Rather, it emphasizes minimalizing the impact of disease-related factors on the occupational behaviour of the individual, and making adjustments in lifestyle and task performance in order to accommodate to limitations and maximize remaining potentials.

Each therapist will want to phrase her/his own description in order to be comfortable with the sentiments that it expresses and to be confident about the fulfilment of the commitments that it includes.

Pre-assessment Considerations

Kielhofner (1985, p. 137) described the pre-assessment phase of assessment as 'identification of clinical questions'. This initial process is very important in working with people who have multiple problems. Clues to these questions may be found in the initial referral or from colleagues who have already met the individual. From this pre-assessment work a basic, flexible plan for the assessment can be formulated, and any appropriate tools and equipment prepared. The pre-assessment information gathering will include the problems that might be experienced in relating to a person who is angry, in denial or depressed. Here the occupational therapist has the advantage of a generic training that allows access to strategies learnt in the mental health field. If the person is at this stage of her/his MS, it may be most effective to concentrate on a problem that the individual identifies as important, which is also soluble. This should allow a relationship of trust to begin to be developed before the assessment of other activities is undertaken.

Staples and Lincoln (1979) and Lincoln (1981) described a problem presented by people with MS who have intellectual deficits. These people can appear capable but give unrealistic reports of their own abilities in activities of daily living. Lincoln (1981) describes the need to seek corroborative evidence from a relative or an occupational therapist. For the occupational therapist it is essential to observe the performance of the necessary activities. Often people with this sort of intellectual deficit can converse rationally and say that they are coping but do not perform activities when requested although they do not have any obvious physical limitations. Their problems are difficult to identify without practical observation, and present difficult problems for the family.

There are currently several generalizations about people with MS, and the factors that indicate the course of their disease, for example there is speculation about a relationship between age of onset and the speed of progress of the disease. Few of these speculations have any evidential basis. One that does have such credibility is cited in Chapter 1: that rapid cognitive deterioration tends to follow in a person who presents with severe ataxia (Mendez, 1995). It is therefore particularly important to build a strong rapport with people who do present with severe ataxia as this may facilitate ongoing intervention and support should cognitive deterioration occur.

Standard Assessments and Tools

All occupational therapy assessments will require a written record of the process and possibly the completion of standardized measurement scales. However, it is important to remember that a person who has recently been referred may have met several professionals within a fairly short period of time and been asked for the same basic personal information each time. This repetition may produce attitudes ranging from mild frustration to an angry assertion that valuable time is being wasted. It is of course vital to establish that the person being interviewed is the one who was referred but basic data can usually be obtained centrally. In explaining to the person that this information has already been acquired it will be necessary to deal with the question 'do you all talk about me?' It is important that people are aware of the amount of liaison that takes place within the multidisciplinary team and how staff can access group opinions and input their own requirements and opinions.

The initial assessment is a two-way process, where the occupational therapist collects the information that has been identified as potentially useful, and the patient explains the impact of the current symptoms on his/her daily life. This interview may be purely verbal or standardized measurement scales can be used. There are currently very few standard measures that have been validated specifically for people who have MS, although guidelines will be available from the College of Occupational Therapists in the future, following a national (UK) study under way at present. There are also reservations about the use of standard assessments; some occupational therapists feel that they tend to distract from the individuality of the person being assessed (Foster, 1996). They should never be followed slavishly, especially if it becomes obvious that the data are irrelevant to the person's situation and problems, or if the process is causing distress. Also, because of the variable nature of MS an assessment score may only be valid under the conditions in which it is made. A person's ability may vary with the time of day, the ambient temperature and his/her general state of health.

However, these assessments are important for a number of reasons:

- A standard measure can be repeated and will serve as an indicator of change in the person's skills or activities. For people with MS, no change may represent a successful outcome.
- Treatment goals set with the patient are required to be measurable; therefore for some goals a measurable scale is necessary.
- If used nationally, therapists can pass on information, with the person's permission, should he/she move house. Equally the person can move about the country and not have to go through a lot of explanations at each new hospital.
- Completing a standard measure ensures that all areas of the assessment are investigated.
- Widely used, standard measures can be useful for research.

Most assessments are used as outcome measures to evaluate the agreed treatment. This is effective for people who have been in an MS relapse and are regaining function but for people with progressive disease the goal may be to maintain their present level of skill. Clearly the number of assessments mentioned in this and subsequent chapters could not be undertaken in one interview session, and not even in one average inpatient admission, and not all are relevant to each individual. The choice of tools should be guided by the initial referral, the identification of clinical questions and subsequently by problems as they are presented by the patient or observed by staff. In some areas of occupational therapy a final assessment is appropriate; this is not the case for people with MS, although standard measures used in the initial assessment may be repeated at the end of a period of intervention to provide evidence of outcome. However, there is no final stage for a person with MS. Ongoing, occasional contact is the ideal, with the certainty for the person that new problems can be presented as they arise.

For people with MS, the areas for which standard measures can be used include activities of daily living, cognitive and perceptual awareness, and physical condition including pain, sensation, muscle strength, ataxia, spasticity and upper limb dexterity. Other valuable investigations include role, sexuality and health locus of control. Work, fatigue, leisure, mobility and the domestic environment are considered in later chapters. Where possible the assessment of ataxia, muscle strength, range of movement and spasticity are most effective in joint assessment with a physiotherapist.

Measurement of Activities of Daily Living (ADL)

Katz Index of ADL (Katz et al., 1963)

The Katz index evaluates six functions; scoring is based on the developmental sequence of self-care skills, in the belief that these return in a predictable order after disease or trauma. Feeding is the most basic function followed by continence, transfers, going to the toilet, dressing and bathing. Scoring indicates how many functions the patient can perform independently. Although once the most frequently used scale, Wade (1992) describes the Bartel Index as now superior.

The Bartel Index (Mahoney and Bartel, 1965)

This was found by Wade (1992) to be the measure most frequently used, among a wide range of others. It is considered by its authors to be a measure of independence, with scores for the individual items being more meaningful than the total score. They accepted that this scale did not reflect the whole of necessary human activity. For a person who receives the maximum score on the Bartel Index, 'this does not mean that he is able to live alone: he may not be able to cook, keep house and meet the public, but he is able to get along without attendant care' (Mahoney and Bartel 1965, p. 62). Although the most widely used scale, the Bartel Index has been criticized for being insensitive with only one category between fully dependent and fully independent. Therefore a modified version was designed (Shah et al., 1989).

The Modified Bartel Index (Shah, 1998)

This introduced a five-point scoring plan for the 10 domains of the Bartel Index, which increased the sensitivity of the scale. These are: 1 = unable to perform, 2 = substantial help required, 3 = moderate help required, 4 = minimal help required, 5 = fully independent. The activities are also weighted to reflect their importance to independent living. For occupational therapists using the Bartel Index, the modified version can be found in Shah et al. (2000).

The Functional Independence Measure (Granger et al., 1986)

More recently measures have been designed that are intended to investigate a broader spectrum of activities of daily living. The best documented of these is the Functional Independence Measure (FIM). This is in regular use in some areas of health care, well supported by an instruction manual and training courses. It is being revalidated in some countries where the use of language differs enough to make the original versions questionable. The Functional Independence Measure uses a seven-point scale to evaluate the well-known activities of daily living with communication and social cognition added. It is designed to be a measure of disability and therefore useful in rehabilitation where team programmes include joint assessment and evaluation. Some rehabilitation teams find it too time consuming to be practical in regular use.

Measurement of Cognition

Cognition refers to the ability of the brain to process, store, retrieve and manipulate information (Prigadano and Fordyce, 1986). The processes that can be measured by occupational therapists are attention, orientation, problem solving and memory. A baseline assessment of these processes may be enough information in most instances. As some people with MS may find the tests demeaning it is recommended that a basic screening test is known to be standard practice. Individuals will not then feel that they have been selected as appearing to have problems. Three measurement tools are described, beginning with a basic screening test, followed by a specific test of memory and finally a more complex and expensive cognitive assessment that covers more aspects of cognition.

Basic screening: the Mini-Mental State Examination (MMSE) (Folstein et al., 1975)

This is a quick, simple, cognitive screening test. Dick (1984) found it to be a quick and valuable test for simple bedside screening, for serial assessment of cognitive function. He found that its scores do not appear to be influenced by repeated applications, but it seemed to be vulnerable to the effects of age, education and socioeconomic status. The score below which people are considered to have cognitive problems was originally between 20 and 21 out of 30 (Folstein et al., 1975). Dick (1984) increased this to between 23 and 24, although he noted that this could misclassify people of low educational achievement. This figure was questioned by Hodges

(1994) who offered the scores of 29 for people in their forties and 28 for those in their fifties and sixties. Wade (1992) offered a different approach to the information gathered from the MMSE, and suggested that it was important to study the individual responses to the questions rather than the total score.

Memory testing: the Rivermead Behavioural Memory Test (Wilson et al., 1985, 1989)

Memory is a cognitive function that is undoubtedly affected by MS; other cognitive functions are more debatable. It is common for people with MS to ask to have a memory test, because they are forgetting things and possibly in the hope of reassurance. The Rivermead Behavioural Memory Test is used to test recall, both immediate and after an interval. It tests recognition of faces from photographs and objects from line drawings, also recall of the salient points of a short passage of prose, and following a route around the environment after it has first been demonstrated to the individual concerned. The scoring form for the test explains how to score the patient's responses and the manual describes the meaning of the scores. The test can be repeated without retest problems because the box contains several versions of each test item. It is not expensive and details of the UK supplier can be found in Chapter 11. For use with a person who is mobilizing in a wheelchair the occupational therapist should also use one when demonstrating the 'route', or at least be certain that the 'route' is wheelchair negotiable. If this is not done the patient may be required to do something that has not been demonstrated to him/her, which may confuse him/her and lead to distracting conversation.

Measurement of cognition: the Cognitive Assessment of Minnesota (Rustad et al., 1993)

Other cognitive problems that arise are not so easy to identify in MS as in, for example, stroke. The individual, her/his family and professionals may suspect that there is a cognitive problem but isolating discrete problems is not easy. The test currently offering the best results is the Cognitive Assessment of Minnesota. This test was actually developed by occupational therapists, for use with adults. It consists of 17 subtests, testing attention, orientation, problem solving and abstract reasoning. The address for information about this test in the UK can be found in Chapter 11.

Measurement of Perception

Perception refers to the integration of sensory impressions into psychologically meaningful information (Lezak, 1976). Often in MS perceptual problems occur in the later stages of the disease and are accompanied by a form of dementia. Visual acuity is also a problem both in the process of perception and in the use of the tests that need intact vision to provide accurate results. The perceptual problems that can be present in MS include apraxia of the limb(s), construction and dressing, left/right discrimination, figure–ground discrimination, body awareness and spatial relations. Each of these will be described briefly, and possible tests suggested. There is no one set of test material that includes assessments for all of these; some are available in the Rivermead Perceptual Assessment Battery (Barer et al., 1990) and in the more male-orientated Chessington Occupational Therapy Neurological Assessment Battery (COTNAB).

Limb apraxia can take either of two forms: ideomotor, where spontaneous acts can be achieved but verbal instructions cannot be followed, and ideational, where difficulty is experienced in sequencing motor activities. Informally, assessment can be part of PADL sessions; formal assessment involves asking the person to perform various activities – for example combing the hair. A list of these activities, with advice on conducting them and their interpretation can be found in Quintana (1995, pp. 212–213)

Construction apraxia is the inability to place three-dimensional objects in space. It tends to be conceived as building with wooden blocks, but for the occupational therapist it is more helpful to imagine it as setting a table or preparing vegetables. This is a daily living activity where specific items have an assigned place, possibly with cultural meaning. In these terms it can be tested practically during an ADL session.

Dressing apraxia is the inability to put on garments, not being able to tell top from bottom, back from front, or to work out what to do with sleeves. It usually occurs in the later stages of MS, but can be apparent in people who can converse normally and appear superficially to be coping well. It is only apparent in PADL sessions, and only becomes real for other professionals if the person is required to undress for treatment sessions.

Left/right discrimination, when severe, causes presentational problems for the professionals who have to reword treatment instructions to achieve laterality without the words left and right. A light touch accompanied by 'this arm' may be the safest solution. A comprehensive list of activities to test for left/right discrimination can be found in Quintana (1995, p. 207).

Figure–ground discrimination is the ability to see individual objects against a normally confused background. The most frightening manifestation of this problem is missing traffic lights in a busy street. A basic assessment can be achieved, for people with normal visual acuity, by showing outline drawings of everyday items superimposed upon each other, and asking the person to name each one. For a person with visual problems a tray of large items mixed together can be effective.

Body awareness is having the concept of one's own body, how it works, and the name and function for each part. It can be tested simply by asking the person to touch, move or name certain parts of the body, and by completing jigsaws of people and faces.

'*Spatial relations*' is the ability to perceive oneself in relationship to the objects and people around one. Compromised spatial relations is particularly relevant to electric wheelchair users and becomes apparent without formal testing. A formal test that is not over-dependent on visual acuity is a positioning blocks test (Zoltan et al., 1986).

Physical Assessment

The physical assessment of people with MS includes consideration of the problems of pain, reduced sensation, and disorders of movement including weakness, ataxia, spasticity and reduced dexterity. In MS, range of movement is affected by weakness of muscles or the presence of spasticity. However, if range appears to be affected, neither of these is present, and the person is cognitively unable to give a reliable history, it is advisable to check the medical notes for previous orthopaedic trauma.

Measurement of pain

Pain is a very personal experience; no two people will experience it in the same way. An individual's pain can only be compared with his/her own, recorded level of pain. The McGill Pain Questionnaire (Melzack, 1975) has been used to investigate pain in MS by Gilmore and Strong (1998); it can be completed relatively quickly, provides information about the quality of pain and is shown to be able to discriminate amongst different pain problems. It contains a 'pain present' intensity scale and a pain-rating index. An alternative simple and practical form of measurement is to ask the person, 'How do you rate your pain on a scale of 1–10', with 1 being no pain and

10 being almost unbearable. This is one section of the Royal Marsden NHS Trust pain chart (Walker, 1987) drawn as a 10-cm line with 1 on the left and 10 on the right. The occupational therapist has to assume that the person's concept of 1 and 10 remains constant and therefore subsequent responses can be related to each other. A cautionary note: many people have been told erroneously that MS does not hurt and may therefore be reluctant to admit to a symptom which could suggest that they are exaggerating or 'unbalanced'.

Assessment of sensation

Areas where the patient complains of reduced sensation can be tested and a sensory distribution plan drawn, if it is felt that this would serve any useful purpose. The only areas that occupational therapists are likely to need to test are the hand and forearm. In order to be really thorough all five stimuli – touch, moving touch, pain, hot and cold – can be used. However, as the main use of the test is as a warning in hazardous situations such as ironing and using an oven, touch is usually adequate. MS does not, of course, affect non-myelinated sensory neurons but they are not the sole conductors of stimuli from a site.

Measurement of muscle strength

For the occupational therapist it is only those muscle groups that are regarded by the patient as a problem or those that affect activities which need to be tested. A basic test of muscle strength is the 'break ' test of muscle strength (Trombly, 1995); in this test the person is positioned so that the muscle to be tested is at the optimum mechanical advantage. The person is asked to move against gravity while the therapist exerts resistance. A numerical measurement scale can be found in Trombly (1995, p. 109); this gives scores of 5 = normal, 4 = good movement against some resistance, 3 = fair movement against gravity only, 2 = fair movement with gravity eliminated, 1 = trace of movement in muscle or tendon, and 0 = no tension.

Assessment of ataxia

Ataxia can be observed clinically. If the person is able to walk she/he will have an unsteady gait on a wide base. Usually one side is more affected that the other and while walking the individual will tend to veer toward that side. People often accommodate for upper limb tremor by holding their arms close to the body and sometimes holding one arm with the opposite hand. The excursion of their tremor can be gauged during activity but it is not necessary to try to measure it accurately.

Measurement of spasticity

Spasticity is one of the most common symptoms of MS, and is very unpleasant for the person concerned. As well as being disabling it is usually painful and increases the sense of helplessness because the individual has reduced control over movement. Spasticity is different for every individual and varies with factors that include the time of day, ambient temperature and the person's state of health. MS-related spasms may be either flexor or extensor. Flexor spasms of the legs produce an involuntary action at the hips and knees, mainly involving the hamstring muscles. Extensor spasms of the legs involve the quadriceps and adductors, resulting in straight legs pulled tightly together, and in the later stages of the disease crossed over at the ankles. Similar patterns of spasticity occur in the upper limbs but they are not so clearly defined.

Simple passive movement of a joint or limb can be used to test individual muscle groups; in normal muscle action this movement is smooth, whereas in the spastic muscle abnormal resistance will occur. Often the beginning and end of the joints' range will be smooth and the middle of the range stiff and resistant. The levels of spasticity found can be recorded using the Ashworth Spasticity Scale (Bohannon and Smith, 1987), which rates spasticity on a scale from 0 = none to 4 = rigid in flexion or extension; for use in some research programmes this scale is required to be scored by a physiotherapist. Wade (1992) described it as simple and the only scale available 'if spasticity needed to be measured'. The scale can be found in Wade (1992, p. 162) and Trombly (1995, p. 169).

Measurement of upper limb dexterity

Upper limb dexterity can be observed clinically in the practice of activities of daily living; it can also be tested formally. The nine-hole peg test (Mathiowetz et al., 1985) was designed to be a simple, sensitive test of upper limb function, specifically for people with MS. The test consists of a board 12.7 cm (5") square, with holes in it laid out like a noughts-and-crosses board. There are nine wooden dowels 7.7 cm (3") long that fit snugly but not tightly into the holes in the board. The individual is asked to place the dowels into the holes in the board, the occupational therapist times the procedure and after 50 seconds the number of pegs placed is counted. Wade (1992) reported that 'normal' people could perform the test in 18 seconds.

Role Investigation

Role is particularly important for people who have MS, because they may have their roles reduced if they lose stamina, power or cognitive skills and they will certainly fear this loss even if they are able to retain all their roles. There may of course also be people who would welcome the opportunity to relinquish some roles. To measure the effect of disease on role performance Kielhofner (1985, pp. 412–415) provided a set of three activities that can be used to gain insight into role performance. The first of these should be adequate for most purposes but the full exercise could be interesting and useful for some people.

Assessment of Sexuality

Sexuality describes a much wider field of activities and attitudes than sexual intercourse between two people, which is an area that patients usually want to discuss with their doctors. Sexuality includes aspects of appearance, attractiveness, and the need to give and receive love, affection and fellowship. These aspects of the individual with MS will only become evident in conversation if the occupational therapist is trusted and seen as being able to offer support. For the aspects of sexuality usually associated with physical contact the Minimal Record of Disability in MS produced by the International Federation of Multiple Sclerosis Societies (Haber and LaRocca, 1985) contains a section headed 'Sexual Inquiry' with a list of 13 questions that cover the possible areas of difficulty in sexual activity. Not all of the questions are relevant to occupational therapy because the solutions are medical, or in the widest sense social. However, the questions are phrased in such an acceptable way that the occupational therapist can learn without being too intrusive which is the appropriate professional to help, or whether referral to an expert agency such as Sexual Problems of the Disabled (SPOD), would be more appropriate. Details of SPOD can be found in Chapter 11.

Health Locus of Control

Health locus of control (HLOC) is not routinely measured in occupational therapy but it can be valuable in the treatment of people with MS, therefore this section is more detailed than those above. HLOC describes the area of people's belief about the control of their health. They can see this as being somewhere on a scale between completely their own responsibility internally located and being due to luck, fate or the medical professions, externally located. Testing the health locus of control of patients can be effective because:

(1) Internal locus of control was shown by Esdaile and Madill (1993) to be correlated with a positive outcome of medical interventions.

(2) People who record internal location are more likely than those with external location to take preventive health measures (Wassem, 1992), which could indicate greater interest in the treatment process being offered. Wassem (1992) suggested that information about the disease and about treatment techniques could be effectively presented in different forms to internally and externally located people. She also found that some people with MS were demoralized by their inability to control MS, while others were empowered to manage their disease. She studied a sample of people 25 years after the onset of MS, and found that the internally located people were still ambulant while the externally located people were reliant on assistive devices.

(3) Sense of control has been shown (Eachus, 1990) to influence the relationship between the therapist and the individual. This information, together with the ability to measure HLOC, can add to the effectiveness of treatment planning in rehabilitation. Perceptions of control have been changed (Johnston et al., 1992) for people attending for physiotherapy. It was possible to influence people's perceived locus of control by the careful selection of structured activities so they may succeed and with encouragement take active responsibility for their own treatment. It is also important that although health care professionals approach internally and externally located people in different ways they do not see one as 'better' than the other. Internally located people may be seen as assertive and effective but they may also be more prone to denial. Externally located people are described as incompetent and retiring; however, they can also accept treatment programmes actively, especially as they can be expected to see the therapist as part of the external environment that controls them.

The measurement tool for health locus of control

Locus of control was first described by Rotter (1954), as part of the development of Social Learning Theory. His measurement scale was the first to be used; it measured the individual's internal–external locus of control. He described people with internal locus of control who believed that events were contingent on their behaviour, whereas people with external locus of control believed that the same events were contingent on luck, fate, chance or powerful others. Rotter's was a generalized theory not specific to health; it was used in some early health-related studies but it produced negative findings (O'Bryan, 1972). A specific measure of health locus of control (HLOC) to help in the prediction of health-related behaviour was devised by Wallston et al. (1976). It has 11 questions and uses a six-point Likert scale, which is a little cumbersome to evaluate; scores around or below the mean indicate internal location, higher scores external location. Scores tend to cluster around the mean, the lower scores indicating internal location. The mean scores recorded by Wallston et al. (1976) were 34.48 and 33.08 for two groups of college students, 35.93 for community residents and 40.05 for hypertensive patients. A recent study (Silcox, 2000) found a mean score of 36.8 for a sample of people with MS.

Analysis of the Data

In an ideal situation the occupational therapist will have completed all the necessary assessments and gleaned information from other appropriate sources before beginning to discuss goals with the patient. This may not always be possible because the person may only be available for a short time or may have been referred for a specific intervention. All of the information gained has to be reviewed in the light of the uncertain nature of the disease and the possibility that some intellectual damage may already be present. Assessment scores may only be accurate at the time that the assessment was made – the abilities of people with MS can fluctuate widely during the course of the day: someone who is independent at getting up in the morning may need help at night. This is one reason why, in the hospital setting, good liaison with night staff is valuable to occupational therapists. Data from them will add further to those gained from assessments made during the day and will assist the occupational therapists, who will be required to advise the home care staff or family.

Uppermost in the analysis of the data should be the patient's perceived needs. These must be central to the consideration of the goals that can be set. It may in some instances be necessary to check with colleagues and other agencies whether it is possible to meet some expressed needs, for example how good the person's mobility is likely to get or whether levels of spasticity can be relieved.

Goal Setting

The patient and the occupational therapist need to discuss the results of the assessments and set goals that the patient wants to achieve and that the occupational therapist believes are attainable. This may need to be tactfully negotiated; the level of openness in the discussion will depend on how far the patient has come in accepting the diagnosis. Goals will of course be functional, measurable and objective (Mahoney and Kannenberg, 1992). With regard to measurement it is necessary to state what the desired outcome should be; it is often hard for people with MS to accept that retaining their existing level of function is a positive result of their hard work. This may be even more difficult for a financial manager to understand; where medicare or other insurance-based medical care is involved there may be other written constraints.

It may be necessary to introduce short-term goals that are achievable and that will add to the individual's quality of life, while the long-term goal to which he/she aspires is much more problematical – for example the person whose sole stated aim is to walk the way that she/he used to and who resents his/her wheelchair. The short-term goal may be to perform activities in assisted standing, to maintain weight bearing and venous return. This may be all that the person will achieve but it allows him/her to maintain the functions that will facilitate walking if he/she experiences a remission in the disease, and helps to reduce potential problems of pressure, oedema and osteoporosis.

Collaborative Assessment

Assessments involving two professionals can be very effective, both for the professionals involved and for the person with MS. For the individual it reduces the number of times that the basic information has to be imparted and the length of time necessary to achieve a full assessment by a team of professionals. Often two slightly different approaches to a problem will stimulate the questions that make a significant contribution to the assessment. It is probably most usual for occupational therapists to undertake joint assessments with physiotherapists, but collaboration with nurses, social workers and care managers is also effective. The availability of other colleagues will depend on the specific area in which the occupational therapist works but can include dietitians, speech and language therapists, wheelchair specialists and architects.

It is advisable to decide before the assessment which of you will lead the discussion and give guidance on any movements required. Each professional will be taking notes of her/his findings and this should be explained to the patient and fed back to him/her at the end of the session. Having the facility to make notes allows the potential to record questions that have been generated by a colleague's interaction with the patient. These can be asked later when it will not interrupt colleagues' ongoing assessment of the patient.

Summary

(1) Pre-assessment considerations: the person, the place and the introduction of occupational therapy.
(2) Standard assessments are discussed, measurement tools and techniques for specific functions are detailed, the measures described are:
    (a) Katz Index of ADL (Katz et al., 1963);
    (b) Bartel Index (Mahoney and Bartel, 1965);
    (c) Modified Bartel Index (Shah, 1998);
    (d) Functional Independence Measure (Granger et al., 1986);
    (e) Mini-Mental State Examination (Folstein et al., 1975);
    (f) Rivermead Behavioural Memory Test (Wilson et al., 1985, 1989);
    (g) Cognitive Assessment of Minnesota (Rustad et al., 1993);
    (h) Rivermead Perceptual Assessment Battery (Barer et al., 1990);
    (i) Chessington Occupational Therapy Neurological Assessment Battery;
    (j) McGill Pain Questionnaire (Melzack, 1975);
    (k) Ashworth Spasticity Scale (Bohannon and Smith, 1987);
    (l) Role performance (Kielhofner, 1985);
    (m) Minimal Record of Disability in MS (Haber and LaRocca, 1985);
    (n) Measurement of health locus of control (Wallston et al., 1976).
(3) Data analysis.
(4) Goal setting.
(5) Collaborative assessment.

Chapter 3
Management

An ongoing programme of treatment is considered to be important for people with MS, in order to maintain and improve their function and to minimize future problems. Rehabilitation is 'not the last resort of the wheelchair bound institutionalized patient, rehabilitation has to start with diagnosis' (Mertin, 1994). Ashburn and De Souza (1988) described short-term rehabilitation programmes as inadequate for people with MS. Whilst considering the possible needs for occupational therapy intervention with people who have MS, it is important to remember that only a minority are likely to need help with the more severe problems considered below.

People with MS can be referred to occupational therapists in a variety of medical and social settings. In the relapse phase of the relapsing and remitting form of MS, people may be admitted to an acute hospital in a state of total collapse. Here the therapist is more likely to be accustomed to assessment and problem-solving intervention and may only see a few people with MS. This is not an ideal situation in which to communicate with individuals and learn about their occupational needs. At this stage they should be allowed to rest until it is clear that the exacerbation has finished and their condition will begin to improve. This does not mean ignoring them, which engenders a feeling of being beyond help, it is important that they are reassured that this is a temporary condition, it will pass and that there is a good chance that they will not become permanently disabled.

A more effective environment for the occupational therapist to work in with people who have MS is the rehabilitation team, of which the patient is a member. The rehabilitation team includes a spectrum of health care professionals with a variety of experience, so that it can be a supportive environment where the occupational therapist can learn and teach skills and attitudes. Occupational therapists also meet people with MS in their own homes, where the relationship established is different and there is less support from colleagues in other disciplines. In this chapter the familiar occupational therapy tasks of providing coping strategies and equipment to assist the activities of daily living will be considered, followed by some methods of treatment for cognitive and perceptual problems. Initially the treatment of the physical symptoms of MS will be discussed, because knowledge of these areas is vital to the performance of the basic activities of daily living.

Treatment of Physical Symptoms

For the occupational therapist the physical symptoms of MS are rarely treated out of the context of an activity that the person is performing or wants to be able to perform. Those therapists who are expert in specific neurodevelopmental techniques will be able to apply the following general comments to their specific technique. The physical symptoms considered are spasticity, ataxia, muscle weakness and problems of sensation. Ideally the occupational therapist who intends to work with people with MS should gain expertise in the philosophy and techniques of 'normal movement'. These skills are invaluable in the treatment of people with altered muscle tone and knowledge of them ensures that occupational therapy in its approaches is compatible with those of colleagues in physiotherapy.

Managing Spasticity

The main treatment for spasticity is pharmacological, but there are roles for the occupational therapist in its management. The first of these is in observing altered muscle tone during the performance of personal activities of daily living, while the correct level of the chosen drug is confirmed. Too much medication will result in weakness and may make activities more difficult. It is quite usual for people with MS to say that they 'stand on their spasm', and that they need it to cope with life. Observation by the occupational therapist is particularly valuable it the pre-assessment of a person with very severe spasm who is being considered for the insertion of a baclofen pump (Porter, 1997). An test injection of intrathecal baclofen is used to determine its potential effect, providing a window of a few hours during which any improvement in activities can be assessed. In these circumstances it is important that a professional who has actually been involved with the person's activity or care problems can assess and report on the degree of any change.

The second role for the occupational therapist is in helping the individual to control the spasms, by giving advice on suitable positioning and seating that will help to minimize spasticity, and also general information on the effects and treatment of spasms. There are some basic rules that can be presented to the individual:

- Avoid positions that make spasticity worse.
- Physical activity should be timed to begin approximately one hour after taking antispasmodic medication. (This is relevant to the timing of the morning drug round in a ward situation where a person will be required to perform activities of daily living.)
- The antispasmodic drug dose should be checked frequently, because spasticity changes.
- Sudden changes in spasticity may occur in the presence of infections, a hot environment, skin sores, or even tight shoes or clothing.

Most national MS societies publish booklets about spasticity and its control; in the UK such a publication is entitled 'Living with Spasticity', in the US 'Managing Specific Issues: Controlling Spasticity'. Addresses for the relevant MS societies can be found in Chapter 11.

Positions that help to avoid triggering the spastic response from the muscles are those that will be easily recognized from the theory of normal movement. The ideal sitting position is with the weight evenly distributed between the buttocks, the spine erect with some lumbar lordosis, hips, knees and ankles at right angles and the feet flat on the floor, with the weight taken through the heels. This is known as the 90° x 90° x 90° position and is a subject of controversy, particularly among wheelchair seating experts. It will be discussed further in Chapter 7. Although this is an ideal position for the inhibition of spasm, in is not normal for people to sit in the same position for any length of time. The individual can be encouraged to achieve this ideal position and then to experiment with variations of position until several have been identified that do not provoke spasms. This will allow them some flexibility without increasing the risk of abnormal muscle tone.

Positioning in bed is equally important and also needs to be explained to the individual and practised to achieve an acceptable, preventive position. Suitable sleeping positions are prone, supine and side lying. Prone is shown in Figure 3.1 (this position inhibits the development of flexion contractures at the hips), supine in Figure 3.2 and side lying in Figure 3.3. These positions involve the use of extra pillows and may need to be taught to family and carers as well as to the patient. It is also helpful to attach a footboard to the bed if the individual shows signs of vulnerability to foot drop (see Figure 3.4). Very severe spasm that can occur in the later stages of the disease often leads to contractures of the hips and knees, which make it difficult for the person to be made comfortable in bed. A T-roll as in Figure 3.5 makes positioning more comfortable. These can be obtained in the UK from Kirton Healthcare and the Royal Hospital for Neuro-disability; both addresses can be found in Chapter 11. It may be necessary to reinforce these techniques with ward staff if they are not experienced in the care of people with MS. A reliable route

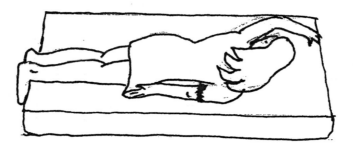

Figure 3.1 Anti-spasticity sleeping positions – prone.

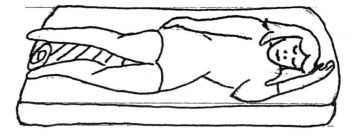

Figure 3.2 Anti-spasticity sleeping positions – supine.

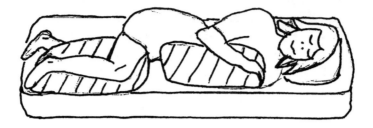

Figure 3.3 Anti-spasticity sleeping positions – side lying.

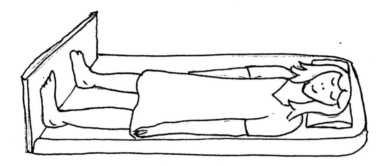

Figure 3.4 A bed footboard to counter foot drop.

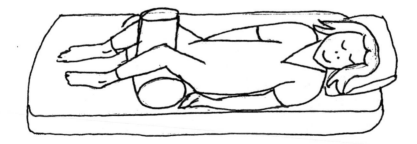

Figure 3.5 A T-roll for positioning in bed.

for communication with night staff will be of benefit to both patient and occupational therapist.

There are several specific techniques that help in the control of severe spasm once it becomes evident. For an individual who experiences mainly extensor spasticity, a severe spasm may result in that person becoming fixed in extension of the hips and knees, in this situation he/she can easily slide from a sitting position to the floor. To relieve this, from a sitting position ask or assist the person to bend forward from the hips, while blocking her/his knees to ensure that she/he does not just slide further forward. In very severe spasm it may be necessary to start by asking the person to bend just the head forward, chin onto the chest, whilst taking long slow breaths. Encourage both the individual and the onlookers to be calm and confident that all will be well.

The difference with flexor spasticity in severe disease is that the flexion of the knees will pull the hips into extension, with the lower legs drawn under the chair, potentially causing damage to the feet and making the person vulnerable to falling forward onto his/her face. Again it is important to help the person to flex his/her hips; this tends to be more painful for people with their legs flexed under them than it is for those with them straight out in front. In a severe flexor spasm a second helper will be necessary to move the feet into a weight-bearing position with the knees and ankles at 90°. A result of altered muscle tone is clonus, that is the regular foot tapping due to spasmodic alteration in contraction and relaxation of the muscles. This can usually be controlled by encouraging weight bearing through the heel, by standing, if possible, or in a sitting position by pressing firmly on the knee, so that the heel is taking weight. In any situation where an attempt is made to relieve spasm, a calm approach and the encouragement to take slow regular breaths will help.

Stretching should be a regular physical treatment for people who have problems of spasm; it is designed to minimize spasticity, also to prevent disability and adaptive changes that result in contractures of the soft tissue. This takes the form of stretching exercises that can be performed by the individual alone, with the aid of a helper, or passively by a carer. These are performed slowly and rhythmically, never using force, moving each joint through its full range of movement, with particular emphasis on the muscle groups that have been identified as potentially causing problems for the individual. This usually includes the full range of movement at the hips where the adductor muscles tend to become very tight, which presents problems with hygiene and positioning in the later stages of the disease. Also, in knees and ankles where shortening of the Achilles tendon is a common problem, this shortening increases the likelihood of weight bearing through the ball of the foot and therefore reinforces abnormal reflex patterns that result in spasticity. Shoulders, elbows and wrists also need to be put through a full range of movements regularly. At a later stage in the disease this stretching may be necessary for comfort and ease of nursing care.

In a team situation the physiotherapists will teach stretching exercises; if necessary they will show the relatives how to assist with stretching. However, these exercises remain relevant to the occupational therapist in activities of daily living, and in the community, where the domiciliary occupational therapist may be the only professional in contact with the person and therefore knowledge of these exercises will be necessary. The National Multiple Sclerosis Society of the USA produces two booklets that explain stretching exercises: *Stretching for People with MS* (Gibson, 2000a) and *Stretching with a Helper for People with MS* (Gibson, 2000b).

In the later stages of the disease high muscle tone leads to contractures of the soft tissue, most often of hips and knees but also of elbows, wrists and hands. The occupational therapist can make or supply night resting splints to help counteract this muscle action. This will aid comfort, the person's appearance and ease of personal hygiene. Splints are most often required for the forearms and hands and are a familiar part of the occupational therapist's skill base. It is vital that the actual people who will be fitting these are shown how to reduce the contractures of the wrist, hand and fingers in order to fit the splint. Night resting splints for the knees can be made or purchased and may be used satisfactorily. Very close observation is necessary with these because the risk of pressure problems in the legs is very high.

Controlling Ataxia

Ataxia is poor neuromuscular coordination causing shaking or tremor of limbs, trunk and head. It is one of the most disabling and difficult symptoms to treat and is most disabling in the upper limb. Medications have only a damping-down effect on the tremor and are likely to produce unacceptable side effects or result in the development of tolerance. Ataxia may be managed to some extent by the techniques of proprioceptive neuromuscular facilitation (PNF) (Myers, 1995). As a preparation for an activity that will involve the upper limb, the person is helped to assume a stable position. The easiest position from which to move on to a purposeful activity is seated with the arms supported on a lapboard or table. Other positions are side lying, lying prone with the weight on the elbows, and kneeling with both hands on a raised surface such as a bench or chair. To help stabilize the position the occupational therapist applies rhythmic rocking movements with hands on both shoulders, or on one shoulder and the pelvis, if the person is in a lying position. Once the individual feels stable the therapist applies resistance to the rocking movements, in order to build up strength and control. After these preparations the activity can be undertaken. A PNF technique that may facilitate control of upper limb movement, for example applying make-up, is to stop in the mid-range of the movement and gain control of the tremor before continuing the movement; it may take several stops to achieve the desired smooth movement.

For upper limb activities it is helpful for the person to hold one hand with the other or to weight bear through one arm whilst using the other. The technique recommended by some experts for overcoming arm tremor is the use of weighted cuffs (Trombly, 1995). These are controversial: some researchers and people with MS have found them successful, while others (Aisen et al., 1993) have not and some insist that they strengthen the tremor. Compston et al. (1993) described how tremors could be modified by relaxing the muscles using comfortable supportive seating and also by avoiding excitement and anxiety. The occupational therapist will therefore be involved in ensuring that suitable supportive seating is available, in the form of either a static armchair or an adapted wheelchair. Relaxation is also helpful in the form most acceptable to the individual; this may be voice or music on tape, visualization or yoga. Some people with severe ataxia find alcohol reduces the tremor, but the occupational therapist may not want to recommend this.

Muscle Weakness
Muscle weakness of the extremities resulting from demyelination of the anterior horn cells or motor nerves is a frequent symptom of MS and there is currently no medical treatment available. Splints or orthotic supports for the wrists may be of help to people with weakness of the upper limb. Normal activity can help to reduce secondary weakness due to disuse; people should be encouraged to maintain as active a lifestyle as possible, within the bounds of their fatigue. However, fatigue is a major problem. Roberts (1997) advised the intervention of physiotherapy and occupational therapy, but

rehabilitation for this weakness is made more difficult because neuromuscular fatigue hampers muscle strengthening.

Coping with the Problems of Altered Sensation

Anaesthesia

Sensory problems in MS result from the loss of myelin from those sensory nerves that are myelinated. The problems include reduced tactile sensation, coldness, pins and needles, tingling, heat or tight, swollen sensations of the extremities. It is important for the occupational therapist to be aware that an individual has areas of affected sensation because he/she, or his/her carers, can then be warned to take safety precautions. These precautions will include care when handling hot equipment such as a kettle or using an oven. Less well known is that a radiator that does not feel very hot will cause a burn if skin is pressed against it for a long time. However, the most important potential problem that can result from poor sensation is the pressure sore. People themselves, family or carers should be reminded to check the vulnerable areas daily. These are the buttocks, sacrum, hips over the greater trochanters of femur, and heels; other areas such as shoulders, elbows and even ears can become vulnerable with prolonged bed rest.

Diplopia

Diplopia or double vision is a common symptom of MS, and is considered separately from other visual problems. It is very troublesome to the individual, making social contacts difficult and the environment even more challenging. It is often treated by the use of an eye patch worn over alternate eyes, changing side each day, or a more sophisticated frosted lens in a pair of spectacles. The role of the occupational therapist is to help the individual to accommodate to this, with activities that require her/him to look carefully to the whole of her/his environment – for example talking to her/him from the occluded side, and seating her/him in a group so that her/his peers are also on the occluded side; ball games in a circle, such as 'piggy in the middle', can be helpful.

Poor vision

The visual problems of people with MS are caused by inflammation of the optic nerve and can take the form of transient loss or blurring of vision. Schapiro and Langer (1994) noted that almost all people with MS have or will have visual symptoms. These problems often occur as part of a relapse when they can be treated by the use of steroids and low vision aids. The occupational therapist will need to be aware of the person's visual status for many obvious reasons related to safety and to the performance of activities. It is also important to remember how much of the information that is given to patients is either given or reinforced by written leaflets, timetables and diaries. Some alternative, either a person to read, family, friend or staff or possibly an audiotape will be necessary. Referral to and liaison with an agency that specializes in help for visually handicapped people may also be important.

Personal Activities of Daily Living

The ideal situation for the inpatient treatment of people in hospital who need intervention because of problems with activities of daily living is in the ward situation. Actually facilitating a person as he/she performs these necessary activities in a real situation is much less embarrassing for the individual. The occupational therapist can, whilst slowly making the bed, observe dressing techniques, or open the lid of the toothpaste tube and chat about a gadget to do this next time.

Washing and Bathing

The potential difficulties that people with MS may have in washing themselves include weakness of the upper limbs, and difficulty in walking, standing and rising from sitting. Weak hands make it difficult to wring a flannel, to unscrew a lid and squeeze a tube. All of these problems can be overcome by the use of one of the multitude of small aids to which occupational therapists have access. People vary in their attitude to these small items: some may take to them immediately and tell anybody who will listen about them. Others may need to be encouraged to persevere with them, whilst some family members are so used to performing these little services that they find it hard to step back. A stool in the bathroom will be helpful in allowing the person to wash while seated. However, it is not possible to perform the whole task of washing in a sitting position, unless the individual is able to afford to use a sophisticated toilet that washes and dries the bottom. A handrail carefully sited beside the hand basin may be effective for as long as the individual can hold with one hand and wash with the other.

Bathing may become difficult for individuals in a variety of ways. They may find difficulty in lifting their legs into the bath, due to spasticity, weakness or occasionally dizziness. They may find it difficult to rise from a seated position on the bottom of the bath; this may be as much related to arm weakness as problems with the legs. The occupational therapist can recommend a wide variety of bath aids and shower installations for use while standing or in sitting. With equipment such as bath boards it is important to allow for weakness of the upper limb and potential unsteadiness in sitting, which make the sliding transfer onto a bath board difficult and unsupported sitting on a bath aid potentially dangerous. It must be remembered that the person's difficulties may not be stable; people with MS are usually at their best in the morning but they are advised to bathe in the evening because taking a bath contributes to their fatigue level and therefore reduces the amount of stamina left for the rest of the day.

All of this equipment is available from a variety of sources; local contacts and services will vary. For comprehensive information about all the equipment available the Hamilton Index from the Disabled Living Foundation, and 'Equipment for the Disabled' from Mary Marlborough Lodge are invaluable; the addresses can be found in Chapter 11. Advice and treatment need to reflect people's very individual attitude to their disease; an expensive permanent solution to the problem needs to be planned with a view to the individual becoming severely disabled, and this may not be acceptable to him/her or to the family. However, it may be more distressing to change temporary equipment each time the person needs more assistance, as this can be seen as one of a series of steps in a downward progression. The choice of options in this situation is a dilemma that will be considered further in Chapter 8.

Using the Toilet

Sitting down on and standing up from a standard height toilet can be a problem, for which the occupational therapist has a range of equipment that may help. It should be noted that when a toilet seat is raised, unless the person has very long legs, the hips and knees are no longer at 90° or the feet flat on the floor. Quite apart from problems of muscle tone, this makes defaecation less spontaneous for people who already have a tendency to constipation. Equipment ranges from the basic raised toilet seat and surround to the sophisticated toilet installation that has the facility to wash and dry with hot air.

For some people, cleaning the perineum after using the toilet is a major problem and one that they are reluctant to discuss. There is a range of long-handled devices that can hold toilet paper; some of these may need the handle adapted to make it more secure in weak hands. A washing-up mop is effective if a suitably sterile receptacle can be maintained so that its use does not introduce infection.

For people who are using wheelchairs it is most probable that they will use a front pivot transfer and not a sliding side transfer, which requires considerable arm strength. Their greatest problem is likely to be in adjusting their dress before and after using the toilet; this can be alleviated to some extent by the adaptation of clothing. Grab-rails are useful but only if the individual has sufficient balance and power in the arms to use them safely. A mirror to check that everything is pulled up or down correctly is helpful.

Ultimately it may be necessary, mainly due to problems with rapid access to a toilet in a bathroom and space to make assisted transfers, to use a commode. This is a coping strategy that may have to be introduced gently and discussed with both the individual and her/his carers. A commode needs to be very stable so that it does not tip if just one armrest is leant on. If a wheeled commode is used it should have brakes, preferably on all four wheels, and these should be applied for all transfers. There are many different types of commodes and where possible the person should have access to several models and be able to select the one he/she finds most comfortable. Where practicable people much prefer these to be wheeled over a normal toilet.

Dressing

The problems that MS creates for people when they are dressing and undressing are mainly due to lack of dexterity, poor balance and weakness of the arms. There is again a variety of small items of equipment that can help, but they will be more acceptable to some people than to others. Few people find the buttonhook a great friend but often they find that a reaching aid can be very useful, for collecting garments and for positioning and pulling up lower garments. It may be necessary to encourage people to change their wardrobe gradually so that they have garments that are easier to put on but still create the required look. It is possible to obtain fashionable clothes that are cut for wheelchair users (information available from the Disabled Living Foundation). It is important to stress that disability does not equate with being dowdy or presenting an institutional appearance. If people have reduced dexterity or need help with dressing it is important that their garments have plenty of stretch and are well made; carers tend to be quite rough with garments when adjusting them. In some stretchy garments the sewing thread does not have as much elasticity as the garment and is soon broken, leading to open seams and unstitched hems. The Disabled Living Foundation publishes a book about dressing techniques that is useful to keep in the department; the address can be found in Chapter 11.

Grooming

Grooming can be the most personal of all the activities of daily living or the least important, depending on the personality. A person who is not exhibiting concern about grooming may have cultural or religious reasons or just have 'always been like that', but it may be a reaction to her/his condition, or the result of anger or depression. It is important to investigate and where possible check with the family or friends. An attractive hairstyle, make-up or a close shave may make a lot of difference to the person's self-esteem and small items of equipment are available to help with this.

As a majority of people with MS are female and many are well below the age of menopause, it may also be necessary to consider the problems of menstruation. The design of sanitary pads is evolving all the time and some that make life more pleasant for able-bodied people are a great help to people with MS. They may be encouraged to experiment with different shapes, sizes and methods of attachment. Often samples of these can be obtained through the continence advisory service. Many people will have an established preference for tampons and a mirror may help in the fitting of these. However, if the occupational therapist becomes aware that the person's memory is suspect she should be advised to avoid tampons because of the risk of toxic shock if the last tampon of the month is not removed.

Eating and Drinking

Eating involves preparing food into bite-sized pieces, getting it safely to the mouth, masticating and swallowing. There is a wide variety of equipment available to help with the first two stages of this process: cutlery with specially shaped or angled handles, cutting tools that use a rocking rather than a sawing motion, spoons where the bowl remains parallel with the floor. Plates can have raised lips to prevent spillage, or hollow plates can be filled with hot water so that for the slow eater food remains reasonably warm. Mobile arm supports may be of assistance to some people although they are most effective on a level plain, for example using a computer. Most people with severe disability from MS can manage 'finger foods' for a lot longer than they can handle cutlery. It is therefore helpful if the occupational therapist in liaison with the dietitian can suggest to the family attractive food items that can be eaten by hand. There are new technological devices being designed and researched that can spoon food from a plate to the mouth of a precisely positioned person; they are operated by a micro-switch that can make use of any movement over which the person has reliable control. The more complex problems, especially mastication and swallowing, should be discussed with a speech and language therapist.

Drinking is made difficult by weakness, tremor and the fear of spilling hot liquid onto the thighs. There are a variety of non-spill cups available, only some of which are acceptable to adults. The most common use of these cups is for small children, and families should be discouraged from buying mugs with child-orientated designs on. Information can be given about sources of appropriate ones. Drinking through a straw is also a solution; there are a variety of straws marketed, some with non-return valves and others that bend or can be bent. In order to drink through a straw comfortably the cup needs to be raised to a position approximately 14 cm (6") below the chin; stands are available for this purpose but a pile of books is adequate. For the wheelchair user substantial stands, either floor or wheelchair mounted, with a cup holder are available. Drinking through a straw does become increasingly difficult for a few people who begin to lose the necessary muscle function. The non-return valve straw is particularly useful for such individuals. Sophisticated solutions are available which deliver a measured volume of liquid to the mouth, through a straw, at the touch of a micro-switch; information about these can be found in the Hamilton Index (address in Chapter 11).

The symptom that causes most problems for people with MS when eating and drinking is tremor, of both the upper limbs and the head. Weighted cuffs may help some people, depending on the professional's attitude to their effectiveness. There is a possible solution for people who have one arm with minimal to moderate tremor and severe tremor in the other. This is to eat with the least affected arm and to use the other hand to support the head, with the elbow resting on the table, which will stabilize both the head and the arm. Ultimately the 'Neater Eater', a spoon on a long handle with a dampening mechanism, works well for people who have tremor but is expensive and needs to be fitted expertly. Addresses for these items of equipment can be found in Chapter 11.

Domestic Activities: Problems and Treatment

The problems that people with MS may experience in relation to the domestic activities of daily living include ataxia and spasticity, weakness, reduced mobility, poor vision, cognitive problems and fatigue (the latter will be discussed in Chapter 5). Following the basic rules of work simplification will help any task-related problems; these rules can be discussed with the patient and given in printed form as a reminder. The most relevant are:

- Plan ahead, prioritize activities.
- Eliminate inessential jobs.
- Spread the heavy tasks across the week.
- Where possible decrease the frequency of tasks.
- Tidy up as you go.
- Rest before exhausted.
- Use the family.
- Work efficiently, collecting all necessary components of the task before beginning.

Ataxia and Spasticity

Ataxia and spasticity will present problems with moving equipment and products – especially hot food – safely, also using tools such as kitchen knives and scissors, and dusting round valuable ornaments. The occupational therapist will need to discuss the available equipment for tasks such as carrying, safety practices and labour-saving devices. Housework is a familiar routine activity and by the time MS has become evident an individual will have established her/his own habitual methods. These can easily be affected slowly and insidiously by the symptoms of MS, especially by changed muscle tone and tremor, so that the person is spending a lot of time during the day moving about and sitting in ways that encourage spasm and ataxia. It is also important to look at the positions assumed whilst doing housework. This can be done in the occupational therapy kitchen or around the department but will be more effective in the person's own home. Posture can be corrected manually and the activities performed with the corrected posture. It may take several sessions before the person can feel the difference and is able to maintain the improved posture in a real situation.

Weakness

There are some simple solutions to help with problems produced by muscular weakness that can be effective, at least when disability is mild to moderate. These involve the use of equipment, and changes in the organization of working practices. Some suggestions are:

- Push, do not carry; use a trolley in the kitchen and for laundry.
- Sit to work in the kitchen; this needs practice in the occupational therapy department and the stool should be taken home only when the person is accustomed to using it.
- When equipment needs to be replaced buy light items; try lifting and carrying a vacuum cleaner, saucepans or crockery before buying them.
- Have baskets at the top and bottom of the stairs for things to be carried up or down, and encourage the family to carry them.

Reduced Mobility

Reduced mobility involves the person in either the use of a wheel-chair for some of the time, or struggling from seat to seat with the aid of grab-rails or walking aids. In either situation a trolley is helpful to move items and equipment but it is essential to ensure that the individual's mobility is safe with a wheeled trolley. At this stage discussion may be necessary about the possible adaptation of the kitchen to be wheelchair accessible, or partially adapted if kitchen tasks are shared with another family member. This may not be an easy subject to approach but may need to be addressed; the topic will be considered in Chapter 8.

Poor Vision

The practical needs of people with poor vision are best addressed by a team that specializes in the rehabilitation of people with a visual disability. However, it will be necessary to practise with low vision aids in the occupational therapy department. Large labels, and colour coding of containers and equipment may make the identification of domestic items easier. Learning to read Braille is of course an option for people with MS who have severe visual problems, but often the sensitivity of their fingers is compromised and reading is difficult.

Cognitive Problems

Severe cognitive problems will eventually preclude the person from joining in domestic activities of daily living, but while the problem is still not disabling, for example in the case of mild memory loss, some treatment strategies are possible. These include making lists of tasks, putting clear covers over the pages of recipe books so that items can be ticked off as they are added, and labelling and colour coding of equipment and stores.

Managing Domestic Help

If disability increases without cognitive impairment it will eventually be necessary to employ help in the home. This is not always a harmonious relationship, at least initially. A typical comment from a lady with MS was 'you have to say thank you, and they don't do it the way I would'. The occupational therapist can help the individual to make lists of jobs that will need to be done, advise on how to negotiate with a potential employee, and possibly even role play the situation. The National MS Society has a publication *Hiring Help at Home* (Siegel, 1996), that provides advice on all elements of employing help, including drawing a job description and interviewing applicants.

Treatment of Impaired Cognition

The cognitive processes that are most frequently impaired by MS are memory, concentration, problem solving, verbal fluency and speed of information processing. The MS Society has published some guidelines for people who find themselves experiencing these problems; this booklet (LaRocca and King, 2000) would be an excellent introduction for people. They suggest that fears should be brought into the open and discussed with medical advisers, peers and the family. Doctors and nurses will be able to arrange for the appropriate tests and treatment sessions to take place.

Other people with MS may be able to share their coping strategies and help remove the feeling of stigma. The family need to understand that the lapses that they have found irritating have an organic cause and that their assistance, or at least their cooperation with compensatory strategies, may be necessary. Where appropriate counselling may be helpful.

For the occupational therapist the choice has to be made between offering people a restorative or a compensatory treatment programme (Sohlberg and Mateer, 1989), or assessing whether the individual can cope with a combination of the two. Restorative treatment comprises the use of treatment for specifically assessed areas of cognitive deficit such as concentration or memory. These areas are focused upon and activities are designed to train people to improve their performance in them. The treatment modalities include computer-based exercises to improve concentration, attention, memory and speed of reaction; some sources of these can be found in Chapter 11. There are also group activities and games where there is peer pressure to join in, concentrate and react quickly. This process is aimed at recovery of function and works best with brain-injured people. In MS there is less chance of restorative treatment being effective because the likelihood is that the deterioration will be progressive.

The compensatory treatment programme does not attempt to encourage recovery of function but to provide strategies that enable individuals to cope in their own environment. In essence, as in other areas of MS care, it concentrates on the individual symptoms rather than their organic cause.

Impaired Memory

Memory is the area on which most information and treatment guidelines are available. Severe loss of memory is incredibly disabling and makes independent living very difficult. The first help for impaired memory is the daily diary, with activities listed and plenty of space for information that needs to be recorded during the day. The occupational therapist should set this up with the individual concerned. They will need to get together and analyse the necessary activities and where problems are likely to arise, then create a checklist with reminders that are meaningful to the patient. This will need to be monitored regularly at first, if possible daily. As the intervals between checks are gradually increased and the routine is safely established, the monitoring can be handed over to a family member or home help. This laborious process is necessary to achieve regular use of the diary; if it is not done the person is unlikely to persevere with it.

Other aids to memory include the use of gadgets to remind people to do something important, for example a timer or alarm watch associated with mealtimes or a box of pills. Some people prefer their reminders in spoken form, so a set of taped cues for sequential activities can be made. It is particularly important to avoid problems in the kitchen that can result from poor memory. To avoid dangers, of which food poisoning is the greatest, a system of date labelling, colour coding or sequencing on shelves needs to be installed. Compensatory memory techniques such as mnemonics and visualizing a person's name with a picture are not recommended in MS because they place heavy demands on already compromised cognitive functions (Sullivan et al., 1989).

Slowed Reaction and Slowness of Speech

Slowed reaction and slowness of speech may be due to motor or cognitive problems, including working memory deficit or any combination of both. Speed of reaction may also be affected by mood, because it requires sustained levels of focused attention that are reduced by depression and fatigue. It may be helped in an environment that excludes noise and other distractions, also by encouraging listening skills in games and discussion groups. If the person has sufficient manual dexterity he/she can use written communication, both within the family and with regular visitors. Committing the responses to a situation to paper allows more thinking time and avoids hesitations in speech. This is, however, only an occasional help; no functional family can communicate only through notes, although on occasion this might help communication with the home help.

These slowed reactions can often encourage other people to try to anticipate the end of a remark and finish sentences for the individual affected by MS. This is often very hard to resist, but can be the first stage in learned dependence that may result in carers taking over more of the person's roles than necessary. The occupational therapist will therefore need to encourage the family to be patient, perhaps by gauging the usual length of the pause before a response is elicited and either counting to themselves or repeating a phrase silently.

Attention and Concentration

Attention and concentration need to be addressed in the first instance in a quiet uncluttered environment where there are no distractions. When an activity that requires focused attention is planned, the person should be reminded to reduce the environmental distractions, that is tidy up as you go along, turn off the radio, persuade the children to play in another room. To help with problem solving the introduction of a decision-making flow chart may be effective; this identifies a series of steps that are necessary to eliminate options and make a decision. This process needs to be practised, several hypothetical problems identified and their solutions traced through the chart. Again the use of such a chart will need to be monitored, intensively at first, and supervision gradually relinquished to the family or home help.

Treatment of Impaired Perception

There is far less advice available about the treatment of perceptual problems and the available suggestions are a combination of restorative and compensatory techniques.

Limb Apraxia

The ideomotor form of limb apraxia only needs to be treated by the occupational therapist if it presents a problem with activities of daily living. Ideational apraxia, if it presents a more obvious difficulty with handling objects, can be addressed by the use of gross motor activities. The person is asked to visualize an action before performing it, and tactile stimulation – as in smoothing a sheet while making the bed – can be used. Kinesthetic and proprioceptive stimuli can also be built into everyday motor activities. Butler (2000) carried out an experiment to evaluate the use of these stimuli in ideomotor apraxia: she used deep pressure massage with oil and cream, and sharp touch using a nailbrush in a rotating movement on the skin. Proprioception was stimulated by leaning on and weight bearing through the arms and wrists; soft touch was experienced using long strokes from a soft cloth and in self-touch the patient stroked her own forearms and hands. This was found to have an immediate effect but no carryover to the next day; however, it was felt that further research into the technique could be effective.

Constructional Apraxia

Problems relating to constructional apraxia can be treated using the same modalities as were used for assessment; that is, using building blocks to form designs from sketches or models. These may begin with very simple models using just three blocks side by side. The complexity can be increased gradually using different shaped blocks and placing them in a three-dimensional pattern. However, people treated using everyday activities have shown more functional improvement. The activity most relevant to the concept of three-dimensional construction is making sandwiches (Neistadt, 1992).

Dressing Apraxia

The treatment for dressing apraxia is practical, during personal activities of daily living sessions. Inconspicuous methods of marking back and front, left and right of garments can be found. Some people find helpful a tape recording of the sequence of clothes that need to be put on when dressing. It is possible to purchase items of clothing that allow easy recognition of the parts or their laterality, for example, shoes with one red and one green sole marking for port and starboard (left and right).

Left/Right Discrimination

This can be addressed by activities that allow the occupational therapist to stress the words left and right at appropriate times, and can include computer exercises and games where laterality is important. Constant reinforcement is helpful, for example a loose brightly coloured hairband worn round one wrist or ankle, and always shaking hands with the person when she/he arrives for treatment and encouraging this among other patients and colleagues.

Figure–Ground Discrimination

This can be treated with scanning activities and with word-search puzzles, which are readily available and enjoyed by a variety of the population so someone with MS could use them in his/her spare time without feeling embarrassed. A compensatory approach would be to encourage an uncluttered environment. Discussion could identify those items in the environment that are important to the person and are difficult for them to recognize; these can then be made more obvious by colour coding or setting them against a plain background.

Body Awareness

Impaired body awareness does not arise as a problem until the later stages of MS, when disability is severe and there are many problems. The suggested treatment modalities that involve sensory stimulation can be achieved through passive stretches and the tactile stimulation involved in assisted personal hygiene.

Spatial Relations

The treatment for problems with the individual's concept of her/his relationship to objects in the environment involves the rehearsal of the ideas of back and front, up and down and the experience of self in relationship to objects in the environment. Suitable activities include table games where objects have to be placed in relationship to each other, such as large noughts and crosses, chess and indoor bowls. For those who are ambulant, an obstacle course or maze can be constructed, where various objects placed in the environment have to be negotiated.

Summary

(1) Ongoing rehabilitation is important for people with MS.
(2) The physical symptoms that can be helped by occupational therapy are spasticity, ataxia, muscle weakness and problems of sensation.
(3) The personal activities of daily living considered are washing and bathing, using the toilet, dressing, grooming, eating and drinking.
(4) Restorative and compensatory treatment, for cognitive and perceptual problems, are described.
(5) Treatment techniques are considered for the cognitive processes most frequently impaired by MS. These are memory, attention and concentration, slowness of reaction and speech.
(6) Treatment techniques for perceptual problems are discussed; these include apraxias, left/right discrimination, body awareness and spatial relations.

Chapter 4
Work and Multiple Sclerosis

Work

Work described as 'occupation' or 'activity' is central to the ethos of occupational therapy. Kielhofner (1992) described work as promoting and maintaining health. This is certainly true in terms of a classic definition of work: 'an instrumental activity carried out by human beings, the object of which is to preserve and maintain life, which is directed at alteration of certain features of man's environment' (Neff, 1985, p. 78). This definition is very broad and includes self-care and domestic work as well as paid employment. As these activities have been considered elsewhere, this chapter will be confined to the subject of paid and voluntary employment outside the home. Neff (1985, p. 78) added to the above definition of work the fact that work:

> Fulfils human needs for a feeling of personal worth and self-esteem, to obtain material goods, to be active, to be respected by others and it contributes to one's identity. These human needs continue to exist despite the presence of chronic illness and reduced work capacity.

Rehabilitation for work is a task that the occupational therapist shares with the Employment Service. Help offered by the Employment Service varies not only with the elected government and current legislation, but also with the wider economic climate. The general public are often unaware of the full range of these services, and it is important that information is available and that the help of the Employment Service is engaged as soon as the person with MS is able to accept it. A later section of this chapter will look at some of the relevant aspects of the current provision of the Employment Services in the UK.

Work and Multiple Sclerosis

Minden (1994) found that 29% of people with MS were working, primarily in 'white-collar' jobs, suggesting that the nature of the person's job prior to the diagnosis of MS is an important factor in the ability to remain in work. It may also indicate an improvement in the possibility of employment for people with MS, because Scheinberg (1980) found only 19.5% of his sample of people with MS were working. However, it may only indicate a change in society's attitudes to women at work, because 37.4% of his sample gave the reason for stopping work as marriage or pregnancy. More recently Finlayson et al. (1998) investigated limitations in the self-care, productivity and employment of people with MS, their sample was sub-divided by type of MS. They found 90% of their sample to have specific problems in relation to work. When divided by type of MS this rose to 90% for people with chronic progressive disease. More surprisingly they found that 71% of people with benign disease had these limitations.

MS only begins before the age of 16 in 5% of cases, therefore the vast majority of patients will have experience of work; most will be established in a chosen job or career. The fact that the longer a person is away from work the harder it will be for them to reintegrate into work (Thurgood, 1999) is particularly relevant to people with MS. It is therefore important, both for the person with MS and for the employer, for him/her to get back to work as soon as possible. It may be ideal for the person to return to work for reduced hours, with the intention of building up work tolerance and gradually returning to the previous working hours. There may be financial problems with this; such problems need to be discussed with the Employment Service or the Benefits Agency.

Work Assessment

The elements of an assessment for a person with MS who is beginning to find difficulties in the workplace include a general history, job site assessment, physical assessment, cognitive assessment and specific assessments of the skills required for particular occupations. In a situation where people with MS are responsible for the safety of others, for example lorry driving, it is important that their abilities are regularly re-evaluated and that they are aware of the possible need for an alternative occupation or role within the working environment.

- General history will include the nature and duration of the employment, the activities that comprise the execution of the job and problems that are presented. Practical considerations also have to be discussed, such as whether the person has all of the appropriate disability allowances, if the Employment Service is already involved in the case and whether travel to work is also a problem.
- Job site assessment may be ideal in order to be certain of what is required of the person in her/his work and the layout of the workplace.
- Physical assessment can involve the incidence of pain and discomfort, the basic tests of manual dexterity, range of movement and grip strength, also balance and mobility. Work tolerance can be assessed and fatigue levels determined as detailed in Chapter 5.
- Cognitive assessments of memory, other aspects of cognition and perception may be necessary; the use of the Chessington Occupational Therapy Neurological Assessment Battery (COTNAB) is more appropriate in the context of some working environments than for an initial assessment.
- Specific assessments of some tasks such as IT skills can be conducted in the occupational therapy department.
- More complex work-related assessments are the province of the Employment Service; information about these can be found in McFadyen and Pratt (1997).

Research into Work and Multiple Sclerosis

Gulick, working in the United States, conducted several research projects into the relationship between work and MS. She looked at the conditions that impede and enhance work performance for people with MS (Gulick, 1989). She also discussed a work assessment scale for people with MS (Gulick, 1991), and a model for the prediction of work performance (Gulick, 1992). In the latter she investigated a model that described the effects on the performance of work of three given facts about the person, namely age, duration of MS and education, as well as work impediments and work enhancers. Age had a negative effect on work performance but duration of MS had a positive effect, in that people had learnt over time to make adjustments for their disease and coped better. A finding of this study was that as work performance deteriorated people adopted work-enhancers, but these could not totally compensate for increased disability or work impediments. With this in mind the next section of this chapter will look at work enhancers that are defined by Gulick (1992, p. 267) as:

- assistive devices;
- human support;
- personal attributes;
- health promotion;
- personal-environment adjustment.

The following section will then consider the work impediments that people may experience; these are:

- reduced work tolerance;
- reduced mobility;
- reduced manual dexterity;
- environmental barriers;
- cognitive decline;
- problems with MS symptoms;
- stress;
- unhelpful employer/colleague attitudes.

The Factors that Enhance Work

Assistive Devices

Assistive devices range from supportive seating, adapted tools and equipment to specialized software for IT users. Some of these can be supplied by the occupational therapist and some through the Employment Service, often with advice from an occupational therapist. REMAP engineers, in cooperation with occupational therapists, may make more complex, individual devices. (Details of REMAP can be found in Chapter 11.)

Human Support

Human support may take the form of family, work colleagues or employers. One lady with MS said of her colleagues, 'we sit in meetings and as the afternoon wears on they look at me and say "the lights are on but nobody is in", then they bring me up to speed afterwards'. Support is often more freely available once colleagues know what is wrong and learn a little about the disease. Most important is that MS cannot be caught by contact with a person who has it.

Personal Attributes

The personal attributes are individual; no two people react in exactly the same way, so a support strategy that works well for one patient may not be successful for another. These attributes can include the person's skill at her/his chosen job and her/his commitment to it, and belief in her/his own ability. Thurgood (1999) suggested that occupational therapists have the core skills to help people to increase their motivation and overcome their difficulties; this area of expertise could be expanded.

Health Promotion

It is important that a person who is beginning to struggle with work because of his/her disease should do everything possible to maintain his/her general health. This may involve advice on diet, for which MS societies publish booklets about nutrition and MS. The occupational therapist may provide instruction and practice on relaxation, using whichever technique works best for the individual. The support of a continence adviser is often valuable and it may need the occupational therapist to make a referral for this help.

Personal-environment Adjustment

Adjustment follows from coming to terms with diagnosis and the acceptance of necessary changes in working practices and other demands on time and energy. This can include looking for employment nearer to home, with more flexible hours, or work that is more sedentary. Duckworth (2001, p. 7) described the socialization of the general public to view disabled people 'not as individuals with immense potential but as individuals limited by their impairments'. Until their diagnosis most people with MS have thought in this way. Then they are exposed to rehabilitation that aims to make people as able bodied as possible; therefore if improvements in their physical condition do not occur, their self-esteem is reduced. The intervention that Duckworth advocated was to break the cycle of low expectation and achievement. People need to be encouraged to believe in their ability to succeed. They need the 'right attitude, habits and expectations', which can be encouraged by achievements and peer support or a course of work rehabilitation in the occupational therapy department.

The Factors that Impede Work Performance

It is only by in-depth discussion with the individual that the occupational therapist is able to identify which, if any, of these factors is affecting a person's ability to work successfully. Once identified some of these factors may be approached either by the occupational therapist or by referral to the Employment Services.

Reduced Work Tolerance

Reduced work tolerance is a problem that is familiar to occupational therapists. It is well documented and in most NHS trusts provision is made for a course of work rehabilitation. This usually includes a varied group of people with both innate or acquired disability and injuries. The work-related difficulties that will be evident for people with MS can be due either to gradual deterioration or to an acute relapse.

In a situation of gradual deterioration the person may have been struggling for some time, often supported by colleagues. He or she may be exhausted, demoralized and seriously considering the options that are available if he/she gives up work. In this instance a period of assessment will be necessary to discover where the difficulties have been and whether they can be solved by practical means. This will also allow the individual to rest and recover some of the attributes that are described as 'work enhancers'. With the agreement of the person concerned the Employment Service should be involved and a clear assessment of the situation made. When the work-related problem is the result of an acute relapse of MS the person may have become severely – if temporarily – disabled, and may possibly have been in bed for several days or weeks. Even with full recovery of function they will have lost some stamina and confidence. For these people a course of work hardening in the occupational therapy department should be adequate. It may be necessary to reassure the family and possibly the employer. The MS societies produce booklets that will be helpful for this.

Reduced Mobility

Reduced mobility may mean that people find difficulty in walking and using steps, and their balance may be unsteady. They may need to use walking aids and possibly a wheelchair. They then need some adaptations to the workplace, either rails to steps and stairs or ramped access for the wheelchair. The possibility of changing the actual position in which they work needs to be considered. They

could move closer to places that need to be visited during the day –
for example, the photocopier, the canteen and the toilet. Floor
surfaces need to be assessed; hazards that could cause trips or falls
should, where possible, be removed or highlighted. These interventions involve the occupational therapist in cooperation with the
Employment Service and the employer. Some of these precautions
are now part of the health and safety regulations for all workers.

Reduced Manual Dexterity

Reduced manual dexterity in MS may be due to muscle weakness,
anaesthesia or pins and needles; it is unlikely that these can be
improved by therapeutic exercises but they can to some extent be
alleviated by the provision of assistive devices. A clear understanding
of the precise nature of the problems may make it possible to invest
in alternative coping strategies such as protective gloves, adapted
handles for machinery, clamps, non-slip surfaces and using tools,
rather than fingers, to pick up and place objects.

Environmental Barriers

Environmental barriers become evident when the person with MS
has limited mobility or needs to use a wheelchair. These include
access to the place of work, freedom and safety of movement within
the place of work and also transport to and from work. These are
areas with which the Employment Service will be able to provide
help, but the occupational therapist should be available to advise
on suitable adaptations. Although help with transport can be available through the Employment Service, the occupational therapist
may find during assessment that what is required is a specialist
driving assessment and possibly modifications to the person's
vehicle. On their own these environmental problems are practical
and usually soluble but they rarely occur in isolation from other
problems.

Cognitive Decline

Cognitive decline is possibly the problem least amenable to any
solution and often the individual does not recognize problems as
they are developing. Both the occupational therapist and the
Employment Service have access to assessment tools for an
employee's cognitive status. Limited support in terms of memory
strategies and concentration exercises is possible but this would need
to be in cooperation with a very supportive employer.

Problems with MS Symptoms

Apart from those already mentioned, the symptoms that cause most difficulty in the working environment are fatigue, which will be discussed in Chapter 5, and problems with continence. Urinary urgency and frequency are symptoms that not only disrupt working patterns but can become stressful if colleagues and employers are not supportive. It is not unusual for a person to have to make up to 20 visits to the toilet during a working morning, before she/he receives help with their continence. Referral to a specialist continence nurse and possibly advice about adapted clothing will be of assistance.

Stress

Stress is a major factor in MS; the MS Society (1996) suggested that the very fact of having MS was in itself stressful, until people come to accept it. Flanagan (1994) described stress as an emotional response with cognitive components and stated that it was a state of arousal related to the innate 'fight and flight' response of the autonomic nervous system. Stressors can be from three sources: environmental such as noise and pollution, which are present in some workplaces; occupational from the demands of the job or unemployment; and life events such as bereavement and divorce. Stress has been regularly mentioned anecdotally as a factor in MS; Elian (1987) discussed the evidence of emotional stress precipitating or just preceding an attack of MS. From this it is reasonable to assume that mental or heavy physical stress could precipitate a relapse in relapsing–remitting disease or make the MS symptoms worse in chronic progressive disease. The MS Society (1996) suggests ways of coping with it, which include changes in work or relationships and financial commitments, and also practical changes in lifestyle. The occupational therapist can help people to cope with stress by teaching relaxation techniques – whichever technique the person finds most effective. These techniques are discussed in Chapter 5.

Unhelpful Employer and Colleague Attitudes

People with MS report unhelpful attitudes to be more of a problem in the early stages of the disease, when they have not disclosed their diagnosis. Until other people are aware of the problem they may perceive fatigue as laziness or too many late nights. Frequent visits to the toilet can be viewed as avoiding work, or made into a hurtful joke. Once the public are aware of the truth and that MS cannot be caught by contact with their colleague, they are usually helpful. The

MS Society produces a booklet entitled *Employing a Person with MS*; this can be given to people to pass on to their employers.

Help Available from the Employment Services

In the UK the Employment Service currently has a scheme for disabled workers entitled 'Access to Work'; a leaflet (ref. DS4) is available from local Jobcentres. A person with MS who is either unemployed and seeking employment or employed and beginning to find difficulties at work can apply for help. This can be done directly from the Jobcentre, where an appointment with the Disability Employment Adviser (DEA) will be made, or through the individual's occupational therapist who will liaise with the DEA. The DEA is part of a Placing, Assessment and Counselling Team (PACT). The services that they are able to provide which are relevant to people with MS include special equipment or alterations to existing equipment, alterations to the workplace, help with travel costs if the disability prevents the use of public transport, a support worker if practical help is necessary and a reader for people with a visual impairment.

The Employment Service is also able to facilitate pre-vocational courses for people who can no longer do a physically demanding job but may be able to cope with a more sedentary occupation. They can arrange job trials with supportive employers, which allow people to update their skills. There is also a scheme to present a disability symbol to employers who show a positive attitude to the employment of disabled people; this helps job seekers to identify a potentially supportive environment. Some of these services also provide tangible advantages for employers, which can enhance the value of disabled workers to potential employers, for example having their own new equipment or specially adapted tools. It is therefore important that people with MS are fully aware of any possible provision, so that they can discuss its potential value at interview for a new job, or during a review of the established one.

Employment and the Disability Discrimination Act 1995

People with MS and in employment are protected by the provisions of the Disability Discrimination Act 1995, with the provision that their condition 'has, or has had, some impact (it need not be substantial) on their ability to carry out normal day to day activities as long as the effect could eventually be expected to be substantial' (RADAR, 2000). The Act does not mention specific disabilities but lists possible functional problem areas; these are mobility, manual dexterity, physical condition, continence, ability to lift, carry or otherwise move everyday objects, speech, hearing and eyesight, memory or ability to concentrate, learn or understand and perception of the risk of physical danger.

The Act specifically mentions adjustments to the work premises; allocating some of the disabled person's work to another person if the disabled person's disability makes it difficult to perform them; transferring them to an existing vacancy, altering working hours, altering the actual position within the workplace, and providing modified equipment, modified instruction and reference manuals. The Act also mentions leave for rehabilitation assessment or treatment but is not specific about whether this should be paid or the amount of sick leave that should be considered reasonable. A study for the Royal National Institute for the Blind (Paschkes-Bell et al., 1996) proposed 'disability leave', which would be time away from work in order for the individual to adapt to his/her employment disability. This is a disability that has a long-term effect on how people work or the sort of work that they can do. This would allow time to make adaptations to the previous workplace or the task, if a person is able to resume his/her previous job.

The Act excludes police and prison officers, firefighters and people employed on board ships, aircraft and hovercraft; it also excludes small businesses with less than 15 employees. The Act covers three aspects of the employment relationship: recruitment, involving the job specification, the application process, advertising and interviewing; the terms and conditions of employment including induction, promotion, training and perks, benefits of employment, promotion and transfer pay; and finally redundancy, redeployment and dismissal. The Act can also apply to other detrimental aspects of employment, such as harassment in the workplace.

Summary

(1)   Work promotes and maintains health.
(2)   Some statistics about employment and MS are presented.
(3)   Assessment for work includes a general history, job site assessment, physical cognitive and specific job-related tasks.

(4) Research has shown that work enhancers and impediments to work, as well as age, duration of MS and education, affect work performance.
(5) Work enhancers are described.
(6) Impediments to work are described.
(7) The current provisions of the Employment Service are described.
(8) The relevant provisions of the Disability Discrimination Act 1995 are described.

Chapter 5
Fatigue in Multiple Sclerosis

What is Known about Fatigue

Fatigue is a real and disabling symptom of MS. Freal et al. (1984) conducted one of the first studies of fatigue in MS, with a sample group that consisted of 656 patients. They found that 78% of the group suffered from fatigue, and 56% found their fatigue so severe as to cause them to have problems with activities of daily living. The symptoms of fatigue that respondents described included 'weakness', 'tiredness', 'need to rest', 'heat makes it worse' and 'other symptoms more apparent'. Fatigue was seen to be always present but at its most disabling in the late afternoon; two-thirds of the sample experienced it daily or almost daily. In 47% the fatigue subsided within a few hours, and 40% reported varying durations for their periods of fatigue. It was unlikely to be a psychosomatic phenomenon, given the high proportion of the MS population having fatigue symptoms. Fisk et al. (1994) found correlation between MS fatigue and mental health, which they attributed to the disruption of lifestyle resulting from the need to accommodate fatigue, which adversely affects mental health. However, they found no correlation between MS fatigue and neurological impairment. Krupp et al. (1995) confirmed that fatigue was an independent problem in MS, which spans all levels of neurological disability. This means that it can be the most disabling symptom for people who have few other problems. A recent study (Cookfair et al., 1997) has shown that for very mildly disabled people a correlation did exist between disability and fatigue. For most people this still means that severe fatigue can affect those who have not been referred to rehabilitation specialists. Their access to treatment and advice on management techniques can be dependent on the services set up for the support of newly diagnosed people in each health area and the input that they receive from the local and national MS Society groups.

High temperatures are an exacerbating factor in MS fatigue. Burnfield (1989c) mentioned the 'hot bath test', which appears to be universally accepted among people with MS as diagnostic of fatigue. The theory of this test is that following a hot bath there is an increase in the symptoms of MS detected by a doctor on physical examination and as experienced by the person with MS. The degree of fatigue is shown to be directly proportional to the temperature of the bath. Dr Krupp and her team from New York have published papers on fatigue in MS since 1988, and they obviously consider temperature to be very important to fatigue in people with MS. This is emphasized by two of the six items in the MS Specific Fatigue Scale (MS-FS) (Krupp et al., 1995): 'heat brings on fatigue' and 'cool temperatures lessen fatigue'. This information is useful in advising people to avoid situations where they are likely to be exposed to heat. It is also particularly important in residential settings where nursing staff often want people to bathe in the morning before therapy sessions.

Fatigue has an impact on social life and role performance. Monks (1989) studied the social aspects of MS fatigue. Her view of the therapeutic goal for people with MS fatigue was 'satisfactory living within the context of fatigue rather than trying to treat the symptom itself'. She described an understanding of fatigue that was qualitative rather than quantitative. Formal treatment strategies such as 'rest' and 'energy management' for the symptom 'fatigue' may not adequately recognize the problems of the 'tired person'. Schwartz et al. (1996) described fatigue as having an impact on role performance. They found that people who could choose or create environments suitable for their psychic or physical conditions reported less global fatigue and fewer fatigue-related symptoms. Vercoulen et al. (1996) also found that a sense of control was closely related to subjective fatigue in their study group. These aspects of fatigue make it particularly relevant to the philosophy of occupational therapy, and therefore a symptom that we should be trying to alleviate. This suggestion is not however new: Kielhofner (1985) discussed the impact of MS fatigue on role performance and conflict with family and friends, only one year after the initial study of fatigue (Freal et al., 1984) was published.

The first contribution to the study of fatigue in MS from an occupational therapist in the UK was by Welham (1995). She surveyed the treatments for fatigue offered by occupational therapists in her area of London, and produced a list of the treatment techniques used. Following this, Bowcher and May (1998) conducted a small inpatient study of an intensive occupational therapy management programme for fatigue, which was shown to be effective. In a larger study, research evidence of the effective treatment of MS fatigue was produced by Di Fabio et al. (1998) from an MS centre in the United States. They studied the effects of a multidisciplinary outpatient treatment programme on people with progressive MS, and found improvements in fatigue as well as symptom frequency and functional status. Their programme took place one day each week for one year and included physiotherapy, occupational therapy and social support. These results, specifically for fatigue, were replicated in a recent study in Cornwall, England (Silcox, 2000).

Most recently, a policy document for evidence-based management strategies for fatigue in MS has been produced by the US-based Multiple Sclerosis Council for Clinical Practice Guidelines (1998). This details an algorithm for the treatment of fatigue from its initial recognition as a problem, through differential diagnosis and medical treatment to referral to allied health professionals for assessment and treatment. The booklet provides a comprehensive account of the current management of fatigue for all medical disciplines. It includes details of assessment techniques including fatigue measurement scales, a sleep questionnaire, an activity diary form and details of alternative management techniques.

Patients' Descriptions of Their Fatigue

There follow some brief statements about their fatigue made by people with MS:

'Fatigue dominates your life and it interferes with everything.'

'My whole body feels like it has come to a full stop.'

'It seems to be there all the time, you never wake up fresh.'

'If I go to the dentist and have an X-ray, the shield they put on is very heavy. If you compare that weight, perhaps even heavier, to your entire body, so there is a lead sheet or suit on your body, that is what fatigue feels like.'

'I would have wanted to do things with the physical symptoms, but with the fatigue you can't do anything at all.'

'When it is severe it certainly messes up your thinking ability.'

'I can hear what is going on but it just does not register. I can't fight it, just nothing goes in.'

'You are not you, nothing is really real, it is all too far away from you.'

'In severe fatigue "activity" is not a word you can use, lifting a cup becomes a major exercise.'

'I wondered whether it was just me.'

How Fatigue Is Measured

Fatigue is a subjective experience somewhat like pain, and is difficult to measure. However, several measures of fatigue have been validated, and the best known are listed below.

The Fatigue Severity Scale (FSS) (Krupp et al., 1988, 1989)

The FSS measures people's own perception of their fatigue using a set of nine questions. These are scored on a seven-point Likert scale, the maximum score for the scale being 6.3. Krupp et al. (1995) gave a lower limit FSS score of 4.0 as the cut-off point for fatigue. The FSS was designed by Dr Krupp's team for use in testing the effectiveness of drugs to alleviate fatigue. It has been shown to be insensitive to energy management programmes and to changes over time. For example, the item 'fatigue interferes with my physical functioning' could be true regardless of the feelings of respondents at the time of assessment. This scale is used in most medical research but is only of use in occupational therapy to provide a baseline figure for the individual's fatigue. It will not provide information or encouragement to people using an energy management programme.

The MS Specific Fatigue Scale (MSFS) (Krupp et al., 1995)

The MS Specific Fatigue Scale (MS-FS) (Krupp et al., 1995) is a six-question scale that was devised as a measurement scale for a drug trial. Krupp and Pollina (1996) explained the need for a new scale, in that the FSS did not show treatment effect in an exercise and drug treatment study. As the name implied, the MS-FS uses six questions, which are specific to MS. It asks about the effects of heat and cold, stress, depression, inactivity and positive experiences. The MS-FS could be effective and less intrusive than any of the other, longer scales if used as the standard clinical measure in the occupational therapy assessment process. However, it will only give a baseline for fatigue. It will not be effective in monitoring the progress of a management programme.

The Fatigue Impact Scale (FIS) (Fisk et al., 1994)

The FIS is a 40-question measure, designed to test the impact of fatigue on activities of daily living. Dr Fisk's team felt that measuring the effect of fatigue on activities was more sensitive than simply asking people to rate their fatigue. It examines people's own perceptions of the functional limitations that they attributed to the symptom 'fatigue'. The 40 questions are subdivided into three domains: physical (10 questions), social (10 questions) and psychosocial (20 questions), the maximum possible score being 160. This scale was designed for work with mixed disabilities and therefore no lower limit for MS fatigue has been identified. It is a long questionnaire and people tend to become frustrated with it; also, some of the questions are difficult to answer if, for example, one does not have a partner or is housebound. The FIS is therefore not ideal for regular use in occupational therapy but can be useful for people who have a strong desire to control their fatigue and ask for help to identify specific problem areas.

The Modified Fatigue Impact Scale (MFIS) (Multiple Sclerosis Council for Clinical Practice Guidelines, 1998)

A specific Fatigue Guidelines Development Panel was set up by the MS Council for Clinical Practice Guidelines, in order to produce treatment guidelines for multiple sclerosis. When studying fatigue they found that the concept of measuring the impact of fatigue on activities was the most effective as an outcome measure. They therefore tested a modified fatigue impact scale (MFIS), and they used expert and client peer review to make their initial selection of the FIS (Fisk et al., 1994a). They then used the results from field testing to reduce the number of questions in the FIS to 21, eliminating items that appeared to be redundant. The maximum score was reduced to 84; the three domains remained the same but the balance was changed to physical (9 questions), cognitive (10 questions) and psychosocial (2 questions).

Visual Analogue Scale

Bowcher and May (1998) did not have access to the MFIS. They found that none of the available scales was sensitive in detecting changes in fatigue as a result of improved management. They used a standard visual analogue scale (10 cm line), which asked people to rate their fatigue on a scale somewhere between 10 = not tired, to 0 = exhausted. The great advantage of this is that it generates ratio data, which can be used with a wide variety of statistical techniques. They found it necessary to make this assessment at specific times of day and to agree on the times when this would yield the most useful information; usually, following the treatment activity was the ideal time.

Measurement Scales in Clinical Use

The Modified Fatigue Impact Scale should now be the measure of choice for clinical use but research based on its use as an outcome measure in occupational therapy is still necessary. There remains a need for occupational therapists to devise and validate a measure of fatigue, ideally a qualitative measure, which is sensitive to changes in fatigue due to better management and energy conservation.

Assessment of Fatigue

The assessment of fatigue levels should be part of the initial occupational therapy assessment process, unless this has already been done and the form included with the referral. Some measurement scales provided a lowest score cut-off limit, to indicate a level at which fatigue is no longer disabling. However, some people whose scores fall below this level may still indicate that fatigue is among their worst symptoms. These people still need to be considered for inclusion in a fatigue management programme. An occupational role list (Kielhofner, 1985), also part of the initial assessment, is essential. It will also be helpful if the health locus of control score (HLOC) (Wallston et al., 1976) is measured as this can guide the occupational therapist in the approach to the provision of a fatigue management programme. It has been shown in Chapter 2 that there are numerous areas to be covered in the first assessment. Therefore it may be more effective, especially in the residential setting, for fatigue assessment forms to be given to the individual for completion before the next occupational therapy session. Sleep problems may exacerbate fatigue. If these are identified, a sleep questionnaire can be used to provide depth of understanding of the individual's sleep problem, if this has not been done prior to referral. A questionnaire is provided in the Multiple Sclerosis Council for Clinical Practice Guidelines (1998).

Other aspects of the initial assessment may be relevant to the treatment of fatigue. The occupational therapist will consider how the physical aspect of the person's disability may affect the generation of fatigue. Compromised gait, ataxia and spasticity all make movement more difficult and therefore more tiring. It is helpful to obtain a full picture of the individual's environment when advising on skills for coping with fatigue. Where possible a home assessment will be of value, plus a driving assessment if appropriate.

The Treatment Programme

The programme for the management of fatigue should be part of the overall treatment programme if the measurement scale indicates a sufficiently high level of fatigue, which will be found in the majority of cases. The occupational therapist's initial aim is to help the person to avoid either of the two extreme positions of 'I hate to ask anyone to help me' and 'I've paid my taxes, brought up my family, now they can look after me'. It has been shown that fatigue in MS is related to role performance, and it is therefore essential to discuss the following treatment techniques in the light of the person's list of roles and attitudes to them. This practice is central to the holistic philosophy of occupational therapy and will help to avoid the temptation to treat symptoms without due regard for the 'tired person'. It requires at least two one-hour sessions, the first to initiate activity analysis by starting an activity diary and to discuss the other techniques available. In the second session the activity diary is analysed and changes planned. Follow up will be necessary after an agreed period (one month is recommended), to discuss progress and make any necessary changes to the programme.

The approach taken by the occupational therapist when helping plan any changes to the pattern of daily activities may be guided by the individual's measured HLOC. The internally located person may need the written information and some support while he/she makes the planned changes to his/her activities, whereas the externally located person may appreciate more direction. The treatment of fatigue mainly requires individual treatment sessions but relaxation and yoga breathing can if necessary take place in a group. People being treated also say that they find group discussion helpful.

The occupational therapist should provide written information that can be studied at home and discussed with the family. Printed leaflets are available from national MS societies but some specialist neurological and MS centres prefer to design their own. Information leaflets should allow space for treatment plans to be written as they are discussed and agreed. The individual will therefore leave the occupational therapy department with a package including an information booklet, a diary to complete for one week, his or her own notes on the subject and possibly a sample relaxation tape.

Treatment Techniques

The fatigue management techniques that are available to occupational therapists include energy conservation, activity assessment and analysis, work simplification, provision of energy-saving equipment, relaxation techniques, encouragement towards general fitness, liaison with statutory services, advice and counselling and postural control. All of these elements of the treatment process should be made available, but it will become clear during the sessions which are of most value to each individual. This section will look at each of these techniques and describe methods of delivering them that have proved to be effective.

Energy Conservation

The basic principles of energy conservation as set out by Trombly (1995) are familiar to most occupational therapists and if correctly attributed, these can be included in any written information which is made available to people who are being treated:

- Plan ahead, organize work.
- Rest before fatigued.
- Eliminate unnecessary tasks.
- Sit to work.
- Have all equipment ready before starting the task.
- Combine tasks to eliminate extra work.
- Work with gravity assisting, not resisting.
- Use lightweight or adapted objects, utensils and tools.
- Use powered tools or equipment.
- Use biometrical principles, levers, force and friction.
- Use two hands.

Most of these points should be self-explanatory although it may well be necessary to explain or at least discuss the effects of gravity and the principles of levers, force and friction.

Gravity affects the weight of items being moved at work, during housework and leisure activities, and the distance from the body of the items being moved, and governs the degree of this effect. Gravity is least when weights are held close to the body and to the body's centre of gravity, which is in front of the central thoracic vertebrae. Advice can include sliding and pushing items rather than lifting them, and dividing loads into manageable quantities. The effects of gravity are even found in the weight of clothes and of course bags; a few moments can be spent in thinking whether everything that is carried around daily is really necessary.

Leverage is a principle that is familiar from long-handled tools such as jar openers; it can be applied to individual situations as they become apparent.

The effects of friction are well understood in the area of pressure control and it is also important to eliminate them in planning to make activities less tiring. Obvious potential problems can be checked, such as ensuring that all wheeled equipment travels smoothly in the required direction, as well as more obscure ones such as friction between the soles of shoes or slippers and some types of carpet.

To the well-known rules of energy conservation can be added a few others, which have been put forward by people taking part in treatment sessions:

- Get enough sleep.
- Do preventive maintenance and cleaning.
- Organize working space.
- Use labour-saving products and techniques.
- Organize work and errands.

One final point which produces a huge 'oh, yes':

- Emotions – both good and bad – use energy.

This is very important to people who are struggling with their disease and all the emotional problems that this entails.

Recording Activity Patterns

The recording of activity patterns involves of all the activities that make up an individual's day-to-day life; it should include everything that she/he does during 24 hours, without being over-intrusive. A good way to start the process is for the individual to set aside a week during which she/he uses a chart to record all of the activities that have been performed during each hour of each day. When this is completed it is possible to look at activity patterns and potential changes to the individual's lifestyle. A suitable weekly diary form is shown in the policy document for evidence-based management strategies for fatigue in MS (Multiple Sclerosis Council for Clinical Practice Guidelines, 1998). This allows each activity to be scored on a scale of 1 = very low to 10 = very high for three aspects: the fatigue that it generates, value to the individual and the satisfaction that it provides.

Cynkin and Robinson (1990) also provide a chart for this purpose, which will be familiar to occupational therapists (in the UK), as well as advice on assessment techniques and interview schedules. This can be completed using symbols for each activity or, as Cynkin and Robinson recommend, using coloured pencils to represent these activities, which gives an immediate impression of the number and intensity of activities. The descriptions that are given to activities will include the standard ones in common use, that is 'sleep', 'self-care', 'eating', 'work', 'leisure alone' and 'leisure in company'. To these people can add their own individual activities, everything from 'committee meetings' to 'sailing', the 'church youth group' to 'cookery demonstration'. Completing the diary form may sound a daunting task at first but in fact is not too time consuming, as for most people a third of the space is filled with the colour or symbol for 'asleep'. When completed these charts can draw attention to activity patterns that are not apparent in day-to-day living. One example is a lady who describes herself as 'just a housewife': her chart shows a week full of caring for an elderly relative, voluntary activities, which include taking the children to various evening activities, and then Saturday in bed. Often people do not realize how full their lives are, and people with MS often work much harder than their peers and families in order to keep up with them. Every therapist should complete this activity diary at least once and be able to discuss the resulting table from personal experience.

Evaluation of Activity Patterns

At the end of the assessment period the individual and the therapist need to set aside an appropriate length of time to discuss the activities charted to plan and agree alterations to the daily pattern. An hour may be necessary if there are a lot of activities to be discussed

and changes negotiated. The first stage of the discussion is to prioritize the listed activities, and how important each one is to the role
performance and self-image of the person concerned. The following
four potential categories could help in the process of setting priorities:

- Activities I have to do myself.
- Activities that I find important for my own morale to do myself.
- Activities that can be changed and made less energy intensive.
- Activities that I am happy to leave for other people to do.

To look at these in more detail, 'Activities I have to do myself' obviously includes self-care and other activities where the individual has
to be present. There is a danger of this category being too large and
considerable discussion may be necessary to help people to let go of
some activities. It may be possible to relinquish the physical activity
while retaining overall control of the situation. It is part of the rehabilitation process to help people to learn the skills necessary to
explain their needs to their families and to train their own carers and
general helpers.

'Activities that I find important for my own morale to do myself'
comprises things that are important to the individual and it is not
wise to expect change in these areas – at least, not at first.

'Activities that can be changed and made less energy intensive'
needs as a group to include all of the activities in the first two categories, and to be considered with the goal of work simplification and
the possible provision of labour-saving equipment.

'Activities that I am happy to leave for other people to do' are
those activities that are identified as available for someone else to do,
with or without supervision. Once the activities in this group have
been identified and written down, it is time to look at ways of imple-
menting change, using the simple headings 'what', 'who', 'how
much'.

- 'What' identifies the activity that is under discussion.
- 'Who' is available to take over this activity: it may be a relative, a
  friend or a paid helper. Beware of the family who takes over far
  too much, for the best of motives, eroding the individual's role
  performance and subtly reducing his/her self-esteem. In the
  UK this may be the point at which to introduce the home care
  adviser and to look at the services available in the area. He or
  she will usually be able to advise about the private as well as the

statutory agencies in the area. In countries where health care is insurance based it may be necessary for the family to employ their own help. The National MS Society of the USA provides an excellent advice leaflet that includes how to write a job description and an employment contract (Siegel, 1996).

• *'How much'* is important and will involve making sure that the individual has all the appropriate allowances before pursuing it. Employing the person's own children is unlikely to be free, as well as becoming increasingly frowned on by society.

Work Simplification

Activities have been identified that the individual can manage but in which fatigue levels would be reduced if these activities involved less lifting and carrying, less moving from place to place, and if the equipment was easier to handle. Planning and achieving these goals is usually possible but needs time and thought, which is just what the occupational therapist is able to facilitate. Simple changes can be made to encourage the person to make changes to her/his usual ways of working. Examples of these can include:

• provision of a kitchen stool to help make work in a sitting position more comfortable;
• having baskets at the top and bottom of the stairs for items that need to be moved so that stair climbing can be kept to the minimum;
• reducing kitchen work by testing and selecting acceptable pre-prepared meals and pre-prepared items that can be combined to make meals;
• simply being encouraged to adjust one's standards can help, for example cleaning every other day rather than daily.

This kind of adjustment can be helped by peer support, and an occasional discussion group for people with similar problems can be effective. The same principles can be applied to the work situation and leisure activities. Sitting, where practical, can be facilitated, equipment can be provided to enable pushing rather than lifting, and tools can be adapted.

Energy-saving Equipment

Energy-saving equipment is certainly a great help to people who need to prioritize and reduce their activities. The occupational therapist can encourage and facilitate people to identify and test specific items of suitable equipment to help them reduce their energy expenditure. This can include everything from the usual bathroom furniture to air-conditioning systems. The big problem is usually cost; even if people are working and have a reasonable income they may still feel the need to save for the future when they might not be able to support themselves financially. This could become part of the negotiation process when discussing the changes that are necessary as a result of the activity recording.

However, there may come a time when the occupational therapist finds it necessary to act as an intermediary and help to raise funds for this equipment. Certainly in the United Kingdom this is a legitimate use of therapist time. The conversation usually starts with 'do you have any charitable connections?' Military service or union affiliation are good starting points but the bulk of requests will go to either the national or local branches of the MS Society. To make such a claim you will be asked to explain why the equipment is not available from a statutory agency. This may require a referral just to get the answer 'no' and a reason why an item of equipment cannot be supplied by the state. In the UK this will vary between districts as well as counties.

Relaxation Techniques

Relaxation is a useful technique in helping to reduce fatigue and it is important to find a technique that the individual feels comfortable with and can learn to use independently. This independence is essential. It is gratifying to be told how much more calm somebody feels after a relaxation group, but if the person cannot achieve the same result in his/her own home the effect is not therapeutic. Wood (1993) described relaxation as widely used to reduce subjective arousal and as part of the cognitive behavioural intervention in fatigue patients. Remarkably little has been written about its use by occupational therapists, considering that most must have used it as a treatment technique during their careers. Fairburn (Fairburn and Fairburn, 1979) gives a script used for basic physical relaxation in a psychiatric setting. This may be too physically based for use with people who may not have full control of their bodies. Jackson (1991) made a small-scale evaluation of the Mitchell Method of Simple Relaxation (1977) and concluded that it had some value in the reduction of tension for people with rheumatoid arthritis. People with MS have also said that they found it useful. There are numerous relaxation tapes and CDs available, ranging from those specifically designed for people with MS to relaxing music and whale song. It is useful to have a small supply of these in the department both to lend to patients and to aid staff confidence in using the technique.

For those who have difficulty with relaxation as a technique, an alternative is yogic breathing. This has the advantage of being possible for people with almost all levels of disability from MS, even those who are immobile in a wheelchair. A script for yogic breathing exercises can be found in virtually any yoga book. Wood (1993) studied the relative effects of relaxation, visualization and yoga, as part of a study of their effects on perceived energy and positive mood. Wood used a group of 'normal' people, but as the purpose of the relaxation techniques being studied was to increase subjective perception of mental and physical energy it was felt that the results were helpful to people with chronic fatigue. She found that, for her subject population, the group who used yogic breathing were the most enthusiastic about its effects. The combination of visualization and relaxation made them feel more sluggish, relaxation and yogic breathing made them more content, and relaxation had the most calming effect. She concluded that a 30-minute session of yoga stretching and breathing exercises produced a marked improvement in perceptions of physical and mental energy.

Temperature Control

Because heat increases fatigue it is helpful if people have strategies to control their body temperature and that of their environment. Personal temperature can be aided by cooling garments and neck or head bands, which are manufactured for use in sporting activities and can be purchased from specialist sports shops. On rare occasions in the UK people may need air conditioning to aid their fatigue, and it is possible that the statutory authorities or the MS societies will help with funding of this. People may need to be advised to give up activities that make fatigue worse, such as sunbathing, travelling in a hot car, and bathing in the morning. They should be advised to carry cool wipes, think carefully about their clothing, and have an umbrella that doubles as a sunshade.

Information and Advice

It is vitally important that people with MS are offered information about all aspects of their disease, but the need for advice will depend on how experienced the individual is. Some people will know exactly what to expect from their fatigue, when it is at its most severe and its effects upon their lives. Others may not have learnt about it or have come to accept it as a real symptom. In the latter case it will be necessary to reassure the person and to explain the reality of the symptom. The occupational therapist needs to be aware of the facts of fatigue and its impact on people's lives. Although fatigue affects individuals to different extents and in different ways, there are some questions that are asked regularly. It is therefore helpful to have standard information available, either from the national MS Society or produced in the occupational therapy department. As visual problems are common in MS it is helpful to have large-print versions of the information, if necessary to read it to people, and to make sure that a friend or family member can re-read it.

The common problems for which advice may be helpful can be set out in the treatment booklet, with some of the solutions that have been suggested by both people with fatigue and researchers. Examples of potential problems are sleep disturbance and sensitivity to heat. Fatigue may be exacerbated by difficulties with sleep, which may be disturbed by involuntary muscle actions 'spasms', or by the need to go to the toilet. In both cases medication or simple exercises may help. Love-making may be frustrating and not lead to restful sleep; the courage to talk about it, counselling, equipment and medication may help.

The stress associated with fatigue may be reduced by support in the form of counselling and support networks from the MS Society. Counselling is a term that is too widely used and should be approached with great caution. It is not simply the giving of advice and a two-day course does not qualify anyone to undertake a potentially demanding technique. Some occupational therapists are accredited counsellors and find that their skills are particularly useful in this area of practice.

Liaison with Statutory Services

The statutory services in this context are most likely to be social work services and the Employment Service. Home adaptations such as bath aids and stair lifts may help to reduce fatigue levels. Some help may be available with the purchase of energy-saving equipment and practical home help may be available. The employment services are able to offer advice, in some instances intercession with employers, and help with adaptations to the workplace. Employment is discussed in Chapter 4.

Keeping Fit and Healthy Eating

It is essential for the well-being of people with MS to keep physically fit within the scope of their abilities, and it helps their fatigue levels. Giving up smoking, maintaining a reasonable weight and following a sensible diet are important. These things can be encouraged by providing information, by poster campaigns and by department-based initiatives such as group talks about sensible diet or even sponsored slimming. A regular exercise programme will help people to become and stay fit. Exercises must not be overdone, but can be followed by a short rest or undertaken in several short sessions during the day. Swimming, yoga and callisthenics are also useful. Aerobic exercises have been shown to be effective in reducing fatigue but should be left to physiotherapy colleagues, unless you are an expert. Most of the people seen by occupational therapists will also have an individually designed physiotherapy programme. Some people also find that exercise helps to relieve muscle spasm, which is a major problem to people with MS and contributes to the generation of fatigue.

Postural Control

The need for help with postural control may be evident at any stage in the progress of the disease. It embraces the assessment and correction of imbalanced posture due to altered muscle tone as soon as it becomes apparent, and also assessment for the provision of adapted seating to provide postural support for the more disabled individual. People with a high level of disability suffer from fatigue but they are not able to follow a self-help programme, which includes the modification of activities, because they are not performing enough activities to modify. For these people comfort in sitting will relieve the fatigue generated by muscles in spasm and by pain. The techniques involved in postural assessment can be found in Chapter 7.

Summary

(1) Fatigue is an important symptom of MS; for mildly disabled people it is often the worst symptom.
(2) The best available measurement scale is the Modified Fatigue Impact Scale (MFIS) (Multiple Sclerosis Council for Clinical Practice Guidelines, 1998).
(3) It is important also to list the individual's occupational roles and to measure her/his health locus of control.

(4) The treatment techniques available to occupational therapists
     are:
     (a) energy conservation;
     (b) activity assessment;
     (c) evaluation of activity patterns;
     (d) work simplification;
     (e) energy-saving equipment;
     (f) relaxation techniques;
     (g) temperature control;
     (h) information and advice;
     (i) liaison with statutory services;
     (j) keeping fit and healthy eating;
     (k) postural control.

Chapter 6
Leisure for People with Multiple Sclerosis

What is Leisure?

Leisure has been defined in many different ways; Dumazedier (1967) described it as having three main functions: relaxation, entertainment and personal development. Kaufman (1988) found that it alleviated anxiety, Dresner (1990) described it as central to the lives of many people and Coleman and Iso-Ahola (1993) stated that it increased a sense of well-being. Di Bona (2000) used a definition of leisure from Beard and Ragheb (1980, p. 24), which would seem to be appropriate to the potential curtailment of leisure activities due to progressive disease:

> ...non-work activities in which you have a free choice as to whether or not to participate. These activities take place in your free time and there is no obligation as to what is chosen or to what extent you participate. Leisure choices can be relatively active or inactive, such as sports or other outdoor activities, reading, television viewing, cultural activities, social activities or hobbies.

In the study that includes this quotation, leisure was described as fulfilling six needs: these are psychological, educational, social, relaxation, psychosocial and aesthetic, all of which have relevance to people with MS. Psychological needs include building and maintaining self-confidence, giving a sense of accomplishment and using one's skills. Educational needs are about learning new information and skills and gaining self-knowledge and understanding of other people. Social needs are for interaction and building relationships with other people. The need to relax and release stress is particularly important to people with MS and fatigue. Psychosocial needs are for physical challenge that helps to maintain fitness and health. Aesthetic needs are about the beauty of the environment where leisure takes place, for it to be clean, fresh and interesting. On a cautionary note Csikszentmihalyi (1993) found television watching to be 'largely unsatisfying' physically, and mentally active pursuits more satisfying than less demanding ones. This finding is of particular concern to the discussion of leisure for people with MS who find their options becoming restricted.

Occupational Therapy and Leisure

Reed (1984) described leisure as strongly influenced by culture and changing over time, as culture shifts. She wrote that occupational therapists should be able to help people to make appropriate, individual choices of leisure activities. Leisure is a part of daily living that has been associated with occupational therapy from its earliest practice. The profession has, at different times, tried to deny involvement in an area of life that could include 'handcrafts', arguably to the detriment of its holistic vision. As a result of her study Di Bona (2000) hoped that it would remind occupational therapists that leisure was a valuable and valid medium for intervention. Therefore the assessment and facilitation of leisure activities is a valid role for an occupational therapist who works with people who have MS. Rewarding leisure activities can make a vital difference to people's lives. Following the diagnosis of MS, when there are no certainties, a combination of reactive depression related to their disease, MS fatigue and other symptoms diminish people's ability to engage in familiar pursuits. It is then easy to slip into unsatisfying TV watching. If these individuals have been committed to an activity that is no longer possible, they may have little idea of where or how to look for alternative leisure outlets.

Occupational therapists have looked at the use of leisure. Drummond (1990) studied the effect of stroke on the leisure activities of a group of 109 people. It is possible to accept that most of her findings can also be applied to people with MS, if some caution is used. Her sample group were older, with a mean age of 71, than an average group of people with MS and their stroke would have been sudden and traumatic rather than insidious and potentially progressive. She defined leisure as: 'an activity chosen primarily for its own sake after the practical necessities of life have been attended to', and she found freedom of choice to be important. The most common reasons given for their change of activity by her group were reduced ability to walk, reduced manual dexterity, poor concentration, problems with continence, lack of transport, embarrassment, finance and the need for physical assistance. These changes in ability cover the whole spectrum of physical, cognitive and social problems. Any of these can be relevant to the leisure changes that people with MS make, and some of these reasons for change are susceptible to occupational therapy intervention.

The occupational therapist may need to discuss a range of activities that are within the person's range of interests and physically possible for them. Motivation can be decreased by the symptoms of the disease and the uncertainty of the prognosis, and some people may be hesitant in making decisions about their lifestyle. The provision of support, advice and equipment may be necessary before they feel able to take part in life outside their homes. People who experience problems with urinary frequency or urgency may be particularly worried about leaving their homes or places where they know the location of toilets. Support could include introducing the individual to a group or to a like-minded person; peer support through the local branch of the MS Society is very positive. Talks on and demonstrations of potential leisure activities can be arranged to take place in the occupational therapy department. A supply of information in the form of leaflets, books, pictures and contact points can be available for people to browse through and discuss with peers and occupational therapists.

One important attitude that is found when discussing activities with some people who have MS is: 'not wanting to do to a lower standard, things that were once done well'. An example is a man who excelled at competitive sailing but was no longer able to remain upright on deck in a rough sea. Among his options were to sail on the MS Society's yacht, or to spend holidays with the Jubilee Sailing Trust (address in Chapter 11). His choice was to work with the local branch of the MS Society and enhance his computer skills. In fact his choices were very limited and involved with the whole fact of his developing MS. His description of the onset and acceptance of his MS can be found at the end of this chapter. It is the role of the occupational therapist to discover, accept and facilitate whichever choice is made.

Assessment of Leisure

For her study of leisure after stroke, Drummond (1990) used an Activities Questionnaire, which listed 37 different activities. Her respondents were asked to indicate how frequently they had taken part in each activity both before and after their stroke. The degree of regularity was measured on a five-point scale from 'never' to 'very regularly'. Although this questionnaire has not been validated for use with people who have MS, it can give a basic view of each person's preferred leisure activities and the changes that have resulted from their disease. The activities enjoyed before the present stage of his/her MS will give an indication of the individual's chosen interests. The second score should indicate what he/she is doing since MS affected his/her life. It will also allow the opportunity to discuss the person's attitude to the loss of previous activities. It will depend on the time available and the occupational therapy department's preference for the use of written assessments whether this Activities Questionnaire is used; the information can be obtained in an interview. An effective method of using the questionnaire is to present it as a group activity to several people with MS. They can be asked to complete the form for themselves but to discuss their options and changes of activity as they do so. Often a peer group will offer suggestions for circumventing a problem and remind people that they used to do something that they have forgotten. At the very least it may assist the individual to lose a sense of isolation and helplessness.

A second measurement scale that can be of use is the Leisure Satisfaction Scale (Beard and Ragheb, 1980), described by Di Bona (2000) it allows people to evaluate the satisfaction that they get for their leisure needs from different activities. The scale describes 51 items in all, covering the six areas of need – psychological, educational, social, relaxation, psychosocial and aesthetic – and the questions can be worded to test one activity or a group of activities. For people with MS the most effective use of this scale would be to allow them to think how their present leisure time is spent and how satisfying it is for them, and whether it provides opportunities to increase their self-confidence, relieve stress, meet people and stretch themselves.

Leisure as a Therapeutic Medium

Here 'therapeutic' can be taken to mean activities that encourage physical movement that will strengthen the unaffected muscles, control spasticity and build exercise tolerance. It also encompasses activities that will maintain self-esteem by using the person's pre-existing skills and her/his place in the community. Finally, it includes activities that promote relaxation; this is particularly important for people who have fatigue with their MS. People with MS are often looking for activities that will help them to maintain their physical skills and do not necessarily see the suggestion that activities are 'good for them' as unwanted intervention by professionals. Two cautions are necessary:

(1) All exercise should be done in moderation; over-exertion can result in several days of immobility.
(2) Heat is a great enemy, and exacerbates fatigue very quickly; people should therefore be warned not to exercise out of doors on hot days, to take cool showers, drink cold drinks and eat iced products. Some specific activities have been identified as particularly helpful to people with MS; these are yoga, swimming, horse riding and keep fit.

Yoga

Yoga is an ideal activity for people with MS (Burnfield, 1989c), it is non-competitive, and one of its main principles is never to do anything beyond one's capacity. It is relaxing both through the winding-down exercises that usually conclude a session, and through the breathing exercises, which are considered the most relaxing of a group of activities used to combat fatigue (Wood, 1993). Yoga is learnt and practised in a group that is usually friendly, like-minded and therefore supportive. The exercises, and especially the relaxation techniques, can be used individually, at home, at work or simply in a stressful situation. People need to understand that yoga will not cure them but it will improve their general level of function. A lady who thoroughly enjoys her yoga sessions said; 'I can't do everything so I go to the back; sometimes I wake up at the end with everybody's blankets piled on top of me'. Yoga groups are available in most areas as part of the Adult Education service. The Yoga For Health Foundation in the UK works closely with the national MS Society, and runs residential courses and holidays; the address can be found in Chapter 11.

Swimming

Swimming is an effective exercise that involves regular movements of all four limbs, in a cool buoyant environment. There is usually an opportunity to join a club and to socialize after swimming. Water is, of course, a therapeutic medium and a physiotherapist can usually provide people with some beneficial exercises to include in their swimming sessions. It is also possible to swim even when walking has become difficult. The proportion of sports centres that have disabled facilities – including pool lifts – is increasing, and details of how to locate these can be found in Chapter 11.

Horse Riding

Horse riding involves physical exercise, the use of virtually all muscle groups, the encouragement to maintain a correct posture and contact with other people and animals. This has been shown to provide physical and social benefits to the individual (Bracher, 2000), and to be relevant to two models of occupational therapy practice. Riding involves interaction with the horse and the environment that can affect any of the three subsystems in the Model of Human Occupation described by Kielhofner (1992). It is also relevant to the Sensory Integration Model, because the continual movement and vestibular stimulation in riding can have a positive effect on the sensory integrative system. Riding allows people to develop a sense of control and usually takes place in an attractive environment. People with MS are eligible to learn to ride with the Riding for the Disabled Association, which combines riding tuition with knowledge of disability and is not expensive for the individual. Information about the Riding for the Disabled Association can be found in Chapter 11.

Keeping Fit

Aerobic exercises have been shown to help MS fatigue (Petajan et al., 1996), but these should be undertaken in moderation and without getting too hot. People should be advised to discuss these exercises with their physiotherapist, as they should for any more strenuous exercises. Details of how to contact sports centres with facilities for the disabled can be found in Chapter 11.

Pet Owning

Pet owning can provide company, affection and stress relief. Dogs can give a sense of security, often allow contact with other dog owners and can be exercised walking beside an electric wheelchair. Those cats that choose to be stroked and sit on laps can also give affection and help relieve stress. For the less active, smaller animals, birds and fish can provide an interest with less effort.

Information Technology as a Leisure Activity

There is a great deal of emphasis today on the importance and relevance to physically disabled people of computer skills. Information technology (IT) skills can introduce new hobbies or open up new employment opportunities that do not require physical strength or full mobility. The age group of people now being diagnosed with MS means that they are likely to be more computer literate than their predecessors and therefore less nervous of IT as a leisure activity. Computers offer a wide range of uses, and because they can be programmed for operation with minimal physical function, they can remain a viable tool throughout the course of MS. A few potential uses are for Internet access, as a replacement for existing hobbies, for word processing, and as a pleasant way to pass the time.

The Internet can be used to gain current information about MS; the national MS societies have sites that are both easy to access and informative. Each national society has slightly different presentations and emphasizes different aspects of MS. Some countries may have access to research findings and certain items of information sooner than others. Contact with other people with MS in a chat-room format can be valuable and may reduce the sense of isolation that some people feel. Home shopping can give more control than giving a shopping list to the family or home help. Almost any other interest can be investigated and people with similar interests may be contacted.

Personal computer (PC) versions of established hobbies can sometimes act as a replacement for the real thing; for example golf can be 'played', football managed, model railways designed and run, quilting and cross stitch designed if they cannot be sewn. Some people will enjoy this; others will just be reminded of what they have lost. Therefore the availability of software needs to be made known and, if interest is expressed, investigated, but only at the patient's request. Word processing can be used for communication and to create a variety of written documents from work schedules for the home help to advertising posters for group activities. Typing can remain a valid form of communication when writing becomes illegible; alternatively, voice-activated word processing may allow the individual to retain written contact with friends. Simply passing the time with one's PC should not be seen as aberrant or stigmatizing; a great many people, fit as well as disabled, get great pleasure from spending leisure time in raiding tombs, playing cards or any other of an ever-expanding number of computer games.

Education and Training through Leisure

Adult education classes are the most obvious form of education through leisure. In most areas of the UK the Adult Education Service provides a wide range of learning experiences, from academic subjects that lead to national examinations, to the simply enjoyable and fulfilling, for example languages for a holiday, art in a variety of media, and cookery. These classes usually build up a friendly supportive group atmosphere, but some people may be happier to go with a friend or even a hospital volunteer until they are confident with the group. Local authorities often offer reduced fees for people in receipt of welfare rights benefits. Education can provide opportunities to learn things that the individual has been too busy to consider in the past, when she/he was enjoying more physical activities or just expending all her/his energy in living and working with MS. People can expand their self-knowledge, pursue interests that have come to the fore because of their disease and learn more about their environment.

Technological Aids and Devices to Aid Leisure

As the previous section has indicated, there is an important role for information technology in leisure activities for people with MS. There are other items of equipment that could be described as technological aids, which include a variety of small, simple items such as adapted garden tools, knitting aids, low-vision aids and bookstands. For the severely disabled person who is an avid reader, page-turning bookstands are available; these can give great pleasure but are expensive and often require practice and patience to learn to manage them well. For those readers whose vision is deteriorating, talking books may be an option. A wide variety of audiotapes is available for purchase, or they may be borrowed from public libraries. There are also talking books for the disabled available from the Listening Library, which is usually accessed through Social Services; the address is in Chapter 11.

Wheelchairs can also be considered as technological equipment, particularly for the fit, active individual who can use a high-specification chair to play tennis or basketball. For the more severely disabled there are attachments for the wheelchair that will facilitate hobbies. For example it is possible to fit a camera tripod to a wheelchair so that the viewfinder is level with the eyes. This may require a camera to which a cable shutter release can be fitted, if the person cannot raise an arm to take the photograph. Similar devices are available to fix an artist's easel and palette, an embroidery frame, a bookstand and many other items. Information about these is available from the Hamilton Index, whose address is in Chapter 11. An engineer from REMAP may be able to make specific individual items that may facilitate a leisure activity.

Leisure Activities and the Environment

Many leisure activities can be made possible for disabled people through modification of the environment allied to well-publicized information about these modifications. The environment in need of change may be the individual's own personal environment, which is their home, garden and immediate neighbourhood. Environmental needs begin with being able to get safely out of the home and into the community, that is sufficiently wide doors, level paths, transport to reach the leisure venue and an adequate income to make this possible. For the wider environment the disability rights movement has applied pressure to make venues accessible and to establish the needs of disabled people. From this movement have come agencies that can promote leisure activities for disabled people and books with an increasingly global view of the needs of wheelchair users and people with visual needs. These services vary between urban and rural areas; most areas have wheelchair-accessible taxis, and some have adapted regular service buses. There are escort services in some areas that facilitate trips to the cinema, theatre, concerts and other social activities. Local services can be investigated through DIAL (details in Chapter 11).

Gardening

A popular leisure activity that can be enjoyed at home is gardening. This can be facilitated by making changes such as widened paths and raised flowerbeds to allow easy access to the garden, and for ease of maintenance. Information about all aspects of gardening, including making an accessible garden, adapted tools, design, flowers of all sorts and container planting can be obtained from Thrive and Horticulture Therapy (addresses and websites are listed in Chapter 11). An interest in gardening can be stimulated by visits to national gardens; in the UK the National Trust has many beautiful gardens, most of which are wheelchair friendly. A leaflet about access is available from the National Trust, the address of which is in Chapter 11. Elsewhere there are botanical gardens in many cities. These mostly have wheelchair access and information about them may be available through Horticulture Therapy. Thrive produces a quarterly magazine to which the occupational therapy department or individual patients can subscribe. Most large local garden centres also have facilities for disabled people.

Holidays and Outings

Information to help people who are considering taking holidays is available from RADAR; this covers advice on access facilities in a number of holiday venues. There are also Smooth Ride Guides that are available from most bookshops; the countries that these currently cover are the UK, USA, Canada and New Zealand. Many people with MS are reluctant to travel to places that they do not know well because of their continence problems. It is not unusual for people to organize the route for a journey based on the availability of public conveniences. If they are not already in touch with a specialist continence nurse people should, if they wish, be put in contact with one. Some assistance can be found with this via the Radar National Key Scheme, which provides a list of specially adapted toilets in each area of the UK and keys to unlock them. The address for RADAR is in Chapter 11.

One Man's Account of the Affect of MS on His Life

At the age of 38 I considered that my life was good. Married, no kids, two cars, own house, and a cat. As an avionics engineer in the RAF working on a helicopter squadron, I had friends, job satisfaction, and fun. I had always thrived in a team of like-minded people with a single objective (putting helicopters in the air), long days, hard work, good friends, *Boy's Own* stuff! All this was underpinned by a brilliant social life, with a choice of either sailing or golf to help pass away the hours. A hard life – but someone had to do it.

At the age of 10 or 11 I learnt to sail a 'Mirror Dinghy'. This simple act was to guide the rest of my life (even now), becoming an obsession in much the same way as football or even train-spotting possesses others. The RAF turned out to be the best place for me to work. In the 1970s, '80s and the first half of the '90s, service personal were encouraged 'to get involved' with what was called 'Adventurous Training', so I sailed my way through life in anything that floated from 22 ft to 55 ft, from the Solent to the Fastnet and from ocean passages to racing around cans. To a lesser extent I played golf with the boys from work two to three times a week.

At this time I worked on a camp in Oxfordshire and lived with my wife Maureen at St Columb Road in Cornwall. The drive back to work from a weekend at home was a four-hour trip (with 60 pasties for the crew room). I started to notice that my right foot would be completely dead by the end of the journey but would be OK within 10 minutes of getting out of the car. Then I found that I could no longer drive for four hours without making a pit stop. As time went on things only got worse, my foot was dead sooner and sometimes I had to make two pit stops. More importantly for me, I began to notice that my golf was suffering and once again it was my right foot causing the problem. I found that I could not lift my toes by the end of a round of golf. This meant that I started to scuff the greens! It was only when I was asked not to play until I was no longer damaging the greens that I went to my GP. After he had listened to my tale he referred me to a neurologist and my life was never the same.

In the RAF you are not only required to do your work, you are also required to carry out Station Duties and, as a Senior Non-commissioned Officer, Secondary Duties as well. With so many extra duties no one liked a shirker. Anyone and everyone, for whatever reason, who was unable to carry out his or her duty is considered a shirker. I've done it myself to others and now found that I was considered a shirker. Friends started to resent that I was medically downgraded and unable to do my share. And the time frame for this change? One day.

Eventually I was sent on long-term sick leave, never to return. At this point I was still on full pay so money was no problem but I found that all I did was sit at home doing nothing. As work was a four-hour drive away I had no one to talk to, other than Maureen (who was brilliant through all of this) and no social life, no sailing, no golf. Now I found myself sat at home, I knew no one, had no friends, no pals, nothing. It took 14 months of sick leave to get the diagnosis and to be discharged from the RAF – 14 months of thinking 'they must have got it wrong, this can't be happening to me'. In all that time my boss, who had heard on the grapevine that I had died, phoned once and when I answered, realizing that I had not died, made his excuses and hung up. No one else from my workplace contacted me; it was like being dropped onto a desert island. After 25 years in the RAF, I can't guess the number of people that I knew, friends I had and from all of them only one kept in touch and still comes to see me.

It was my 40th birthday that this all started, and after seven years things are a bit different. Maureen is now my full-time carer, and I'm no longer on anything like full pay! But I have new friends, other MS sufferers mostly, people I have met at the rehab unit and through the MS Society. But, and those who know me will testify, I'm neither sad, lonely or in need of pity. I have always believed that in this life you either smile with the fairies or cry with the devil, and I've done my crying.

Summary

(1) Leisure is a difficult subject to define, and is very individual.
(2) Watching television has been rated as very low in satisfaction for the individual.
(3) The needs that leisure can fulfil are psychological, educational, social, relaxation, psychosocial and aesthetic.
(4) Leisure can be assessed during an interview by using the Activities Questionnaire or the Leisure Satisfaction Scale.
(5) Occupational therapy intervention in leisure can involve leisure as a therapeutic medium, leisure as educational, facilitating leisure with equipment and information, and modifying the environment to assist leisure.
(6) An account is given of the effects of MS on the life of a man who enjoyed active leisure.

Chapter 7
Mobility for People with Multiple Sclerosis

It has been shown (Aldersea et al., 1999) that therapists gain insufficient knowledge of the prescription of wheelchairs from their basic training. Expertise remains at present with the NHS wheelchair service and specialist suppliers, but can be developed by occupational therapists in specialist services. It is strongly recommended that occupational therapists working regularly with people who have MS should have a copy of Ham et al. (1998), and that they become members of the Posture and Mobility Group, which is an excellent source of information and expert support (details in Chapter 11). The majority of information that is available about mobility and MS is related to the prescription of wheelchairs. However, mobility also includes choice and instruction in the use of walking aids, advice on specialist driving assessment and access to vehicles.

Provision of Walking Aids

Professional skill in the prescription of walking aids and training in their use belongs to physiotherapists. However, some occupational therapists, usually those working in the community, may be expected to supply walking sticks and frames.

Walking Sticks

The basic rule for a walking stick is that when the stick is being used to take weight and assist walking, the top of the stick should be level with the head of the ulna when the patient is standing with the arms at the sides. This allows for an angle of 15° of flexion at the elbow when holding the stick. A longer stick is sometimes used when the aim is to assist balance while all the weight is borne by the legs. Some people find that ergonomically shaped walking stick handles provide great benefit whereas others do not like them, and there is always an individualist who buys his/her own carved stick regardless of height.

Walking Frames

Walking frames should be adjusted so that the person can stand with her/his back straight and the elbows comfortably flexed, again at approximately 15°. A wheeled frame will allow a more fluid and natural pattern of walking, but the therapist needs to be certain that the person can control the frame and that it will not wheel away from him/her.

Provision of Wheelchairs

In the UK wheelchairs are available from the NHS wheelchair service. This service has different titles depending on the policy of the local trust, which provides and maintains a range of basic wheelchairs, and two additional schemes, 'the voucher scheme' and 'the indoor/outdoor electric wheelchair scheme'. The voucher scheme provides an individual who fits specific criteria with a voucher that represents money toward the purchase, from the private sector, of a specific type of wheelchair. The indoor/outdoor electric wheelchair scheme is a government initiative that allowed the NHS wheelchair service to assess and supply these chairs, the numbers of which are limited and subject to specific criteria. This provision is now becoming available under the voucher scheme in most areas. People with MS may be eligible for both of these schemes depending on their level of disability.

In addition to the NHS wheelchair service there is a strong and knowledgeable private sector, which can assess, supply and maintain privately purchased wheelchairs. Some of these will assist in fundraising for people who cannot afford a wheelchair that is considered ideal for them following assessment.

The First Wheelchair

Provision of a person's first wheelchair can constitute a very emotional experience for the individual concerned; it marks deterioration in his/her condition and a move toward the state of dependence that he/she fears. It may be possible to lessen this feeling by stressing the preventive value of a wheelchair. It will be useful as part of the fatigue management programme, on late evenings when exhaustion sets in or for more adventurous outings that have been curtailed because of MS symptoms. Often the patient will ask for 'something light to keep in the car', and she/he may be reluctant to discuss or be measured for this. This approach needs to be challenged because an inappropriate first wheelchair may promote longer-term problems. Some people use and come to accept the posture dictated by their first wheelchair, and if they need to make more use of a chair do not want to change. If for example the seat base of the first wheelchair is too long, or the backrest too inclined (both of which can be the case with the UK's NHS lightweight model), the person may develop a posture in which he/she accommodates to a hip angle considerably greater that 90° and 'windswept legs' (see Figure 7.1). A pushchair with four small wheels is virtually never appropriate, as it does not allow the individual any independence. The exception is where there is severe dementia and the individual could injure him/herself by moving without being aware of his/her environment.

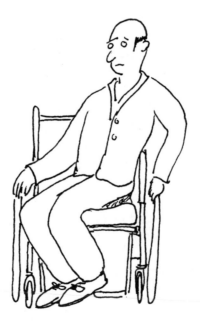

Figure 7.1 Windswept legs, due to unsuitable wheelchair seating.

The role of the occupational therapist in the prescription of a wheelchair does not end with the choice of model and measurement for it. The person needs to be instructed in the techniques of propelling a manual wheelchair, the safety issues that are involved with outdoor mobility and advice on maintenance, tyre pressures and cleaning. The carer needs to be shown how to push a wheelchair safely and with the least stress. The supplier should do this, but it is important to check that information has been provided and is understood. The use of a seat belt needs to be discussed with both user and pusher; there are human rights issues involved with the use of seat belts. Some people see them as unacceptable restraints. There is, however, a real danger of the user being tipped out if a hazard is not noticed or a kerb misjudged. A standard safety belt is designed to fit round the waist and does restrict movement, especially when trying to pick items up from the floor or from shop counters. A posture-control hip strap that fits at an angle of 45° across the hips is a good alternative; if correctly positioned it is more functional, less obvious to the general public and effective as a safety belt.

There is a potential danger in the person with MS or her/his family buying their own wheelchair without advice. Not all mobility specialists have a full understanding of the uncertain nature of MS and the postural problems that can arise. It is possible for a lot of money to be spent on a wheelchair with wonderful geometry that is also a fashion statement. These, however, are designed by and for people with static disabilities who use side transfers and often do not need support for the upper trunk. They may be ideal for some people with MS but not for everybody and it is difficult – and sometimes impossible – to adapt these chairs. The occupational therapist should make every effort to discuss the use of any potential wheelchair with the individual and her/his family. The intended user should be able to spend time in the model assessed as most suitable for him/her. This message can be spread with the cooperation of the local branch of the MS Society, and the local mobility specialist.

Measurement for a Wheelchair

Patients should always be measured, including height and weight, before a wheelchair is prescribed. With the present provision by the NHS in the UK this may seem academic, because the choice of wheelchair is very limited, but it is a requirement of good practice. In order to measure accurately, the person should be seated with hips, knees and ankles flexed at 90° if possible, and have an armrest, either in an upright chair or a wheelchair.

Figures 7.2 and 7.3 show the measurements that need to be taken.

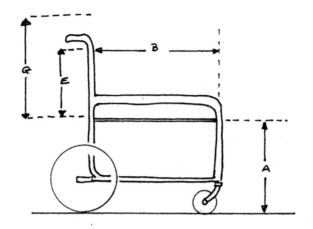

Figure 7.2 Measurements that need to be taken when assessing for a wheelchair – lateral.

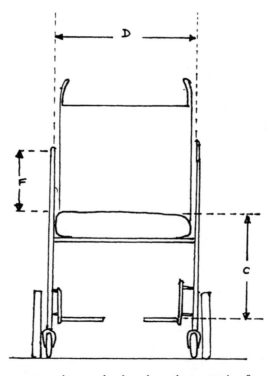

Figure 7.3 Measurements that need to be taken when assessing for a wheelchair – rear view.

Measurement A = Seat Height

Seat height is measured from the floor to the seat at the side where the seat canvas joins the frame. There is rarely much difference in this measurement among standard wheelchairs, but it is important because transfers are affected by very small differences in height. The chosen cushion will make the greatest difference in seat height, and if height for transferring is crucial, allowance should be made for the cushion that has been assessed. A chair that is too high may be unstable, at risk of tipping sideways on uneven ground, and may also present problems with propelling under tables.

Measurement B = Seat Depth

The correct depth of a wheelchair seat is 3–4 cm ($1''$–$1\frac{1}{2}''$) less than the patient's measurement from the back of the buttocks to the back of the knee; 3–4 cm can be estimated by the index and middle fingers of an average hand. When taking measurements for a third party to supply the chair, it must always be made clear whether the measurement is taken with or without the allowance of this 3–4 cm. If the seat is too long there is pressure on the back of the knee that encourages the person to increase the angle at the hip leading to windswept legs, and possible circulation problems and chafing. The individual may then slide down in the chair, losing the lumbar lordosis, until he/she is sitting on the sacrum, which is then vulnerable to pressure. If the seat is too short and the thighs are not adequately supported, the sitting position may be unstable and the pressure risk increased.

Measurement C = Lower Leg Length

This measurement is taken from the inside of the knee wearing average shoes. This determines the height of the footrests. If they are too high the knees are flexed below a right angle, the thighs are unsupported, the weight is thrown back onto the vulnerable ischial area and it may be difficult to propel the chair under a table. If they are too low there will be pressure under the thighs that may increase neurological symptoms in the lower leg. If the feet do not rest comfortably on the footplate, the person may slide forward to position the feet, thus placing pressure on the sacrum. Footplate angle is also important in MS as full foot strike on the plate helps prevent spasm and clonus.

Measurement D = Seat Width

Theoretically the seat width measurement should allow 2.5 cm (1") on either side for the person to wear winter clothes and not have any pressure from the side panels. This can be assessed by passing the flat of the hand between the side panel and the person's thigh. However, if the person is large it is sometimes necessary to compromise on seat width. Access to the average home and to many work, social and leisure facilities is severely restricted if the width of the wheelchair is much greater than the average 64 cm (25"). If this compromise has to be accepted, vulnerable pressure areas must be carefully monitored and where necessary the need explained to the family and carers. People with vulnerable skin should be reminded not to keep items down the side of the chair that could cause pressure, such as handbags, keys and cigarette lighters.

Measurement E = Backrest Height to Mid-scapula or Axilla

This measurement of back height is particularly important for people with MS. The measurement is taken from the seat to the axilla with the person sitting with the arms stretched out parallel to the floor. If the person develops increased extensor muscle tone, this will encourage the hips to slide forward and the back to press against the top of the backrest. The scapulae therefore need to be controlled by the backrest, in order to prevent the occurrence of hyperextension of the spine and the development of a fixed lordosis, as well as excessive wear on the backrest. People with good upper body strength who propel independently prefer to have the back rest 2–5 cm (1"–2") below the scapula but this may not be a good long-term option for a person with MS.

Measurement F = Armrest Height

This should be measured with the forearms resting on an armrest and the shoulders in a neutral, relaxed position. Armrests that are too low encourage lateral deviation and if they are too high the shoulders will be elevated and uncomfortable, leading to muscular fatigue.

Measurement G = Back Height to the Top of the Shoulder

This measurement is only necessary if the person has poor head control and requires a supportive headrest.

Wheelchairs in Permanent Use

For a minority of people with MS the time will come when they need to use a wheelchair for all mobility and may spend most of their day using one. The first essential for good seating in a wheelchair is to have the hips positioned correctly, which should be a priority each time the person sits down. To check position, find the person's iliac crests and place a hand on each, palm facing downwards. It is then possible to assess whether the hands and therefore the hips are level both laterally and from front to back. The importance of this position, which may not feel straight to the individual, must be stressed and encouraged by professionals and carers.

To maintain a comfortable, functional antispasmodic position, the aim should be for an angle of 90° at hips, knees and ankles. This is theoretically ideal but not acceptable to the individual for long periods of time. In an ideal situation the person should move or be moved at regular intervals between bed, a suitable armchair and the adapted wheelchair. More sophisticated seating in a wheelchair may be necessary for the management of severe disability in MS, and this may be vacuum moulded, matrix or carved foam. All of these are only as effective as the original position that the person adopted when the seat or mould for the seat was made. It is essential that the professionals who are involved with these seats are experts, and are aware of the individual's specific problems. The resulting seat should be practical and functional, with appropriate pressure care cushioning. That is, the person should be able to be seated in it regularly and correctly, using the appropriate handling techniques, and should be able to function to his/her maximum ability. There is a temptation to use high doses of antispasmodic drugs just for the day when the seating system is designed, in order to achieve a seat with a good position. However, this rarely produces a result that will be usable in day-to-day care.

It is important that any positioning straps or additional supports should be 'carer proof'. This means that it should be clear what the purpose of an item is, where it fits and under what circumstances it should be adjusted. Not everything can be fixed to the chair, because some parts need to be movable to provide access and straps need to be adjustable in case of weight loss or gain. A teaching session for family and carers needs to be provided, plus written instructions with clear diagrams. These sessions should, where possible, be led by the person with MS, who is the only one who knows whether she/he is comfortable. This allows the individual to practise instructing carers and the carers to accept that the person is able to guide them.

Adapting Wheelchairs for People with MS

Most of the adaptations that are made to wheelchairs are done by skilled technicians, from either the NHS wheelchair service or approved suppliers. Information about the techniques that are available to these experts can be found in Ham et al. (1998). They will have access to purpose-built items of positioning equipment that are expensive and unlikely to be available in most occupational therapy departments. For most people with MS, the occupational therapist spends more time with them and understands their problems and daily living needs better than these colleagues. There are several common problems that people with MS can have with posture in a wheelchair. The most common temporary adaptations that can be made will be described below. For each one, the role of the occupational therapist is the assessment of the problem, and the use of temporary solutions that can be evaluated and discussed with the technical staff.

Extensor Thrust

Extensor thrust results from abnormally high tone in the extensor muscles (Figure 7.4). In severe extensor thrust there will be some permanent high tone and occasional severe extensor spasms that can result in all the major joints of the body being fixed in extension. High temperatures, moving over uneven terrain and sometimes stress can exacerbate this. Extensor thrust is technically best accommodated by a seating system that keeps the hips, knees and ankles at 90°. The most common method of maintaining the position of the hips, a wedged or ramped cushion, can be used and a strap can be placed at 45° from the back of the chair and passing across the hips. More recently the use of a single belt has been questioned; some experts prefer to use a four-point belt. The straps need to be firm and therefore it is necessary to make regular pressure checks, particularly of the sacrum, the ischial tuberosities and where the strap passes over the pelvic bones. Carers tend to want to loosen these straps and therefore need to have the seating plan explained to them. A higher than average, supportive backrest will also be necessary. Once the hips are controlled the knees and ankles usually relax, but on occasions, such as pushing over uneven ground, it may be neces-

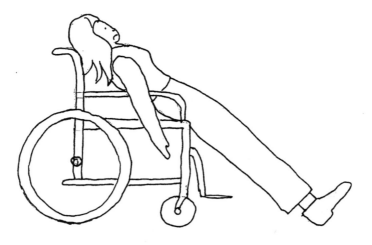

Figure 7.4 Extensor thrust.

sary to control the feet. This can be done with ankle and toe straps on the footrest or simply by bandaging.

Although what is described above is effective and the generally accepted method of controlling spasticity, as already stated this is not an ideal solution for long time-spans. An average fit adult, if made to sit in the same fixed position for 8 to 10 hours, would find, at the least, that his/her knees were stiff and painful and the ankles swollen. Alternative solutions will be expensive: either a sophisticated wheelchair or additional care. The possibilities include moving between bed, the wheelchair and a suitable armchair at regular intervals and the use of a chair with 'tilt in space' that allows the effects of gravity on the position to be changed when necessary. Tilt in space is most effective with electrically controlled tilt so that the user can change her/his own position as she/he feels the need. There is a problem with tilt in space in that the person's orientation is changed, he/she is sometimes not able to make eye contact while talking to companions and tends to be looking at the least interesting part of the room. For the person who is comfortable in a tilted position it may be helpful to raise pictures on the walls, and the television.

Flexor Pull

In wheelchair seating the main effects of flexor pull are on the legs. Once the hips are correctly positioned with a wedged or ramped cushion and a hip strap in place, the tendency is for the knees to be pulled into flexion and therefore the feet are pulled under the seat and behind the footplates (Figure 7.5). This leaves the feet vulnerable to trauma from the wheels and uneven floor surfaces. It also allows for the formation of flexion contractions of the knees. Unless the spasm is very severe it can be controlled by an 'apron' behind the calves, fixed round the uprights of the footplates. The effectiveness of this can be assessed with bandages wrapped round the uprights of the footplates. If the person's heels are at risk of pressure sores regular inspection is essential; a sheepskin-covered 'apron' will help but not solve this problem. Any solution that uses the footplate supports will mean that they cannot be easily removed for transfers. It is, however, unlikely that a person with severe flexion of the knees will be using a standing transfer.

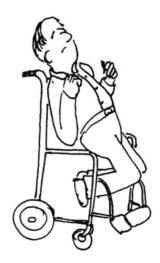

Figure 7.5 Flexor pull.

Lateral Deviation

Lateral deviation describes the person's tendency to lean over the side of the wheelchair (Figure 7.6.). It may be to one side due to abnormal muscle tone, or to either side due to muscle weakness and the position of the pelvis when he/she was seated in the chair. The occupational therapist's first task is therefore to investigate the level of the pelvis, by placing the hands on the iliac crests and estimating any discrepancy. It may be possible to remove the lateral deviation by positioning the person with the pelvis straight. The pelvis is more stable if the thighs are well supported; the cushioning and footrest height should therefore be checked.

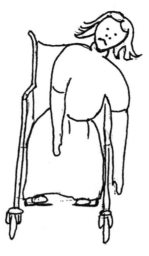

Figure 7.6 Lateral deviation.

If this fails to correct the lateral deviation some side support will be necessary. Figure 7.7. shows the basic design for a simple lateral board that can be made to measure and used to assess the value and potential problems of lateral support. Measurement A–B is the depth of the armrest of the wheelchair, C–D is the height to within 3 cm of the axilla and E–F is the measurement to the front of the chest whilst sitting in the wheelchair. If the board is deeper than necessary it will impair function. To provide even temporary lateral boards, both sides should be supported so that a clear picture of any improvement can be seen. When using these boards the axilla is particularly vulnerable; the top of the board can be padded and frequent checks for pressure should be made.

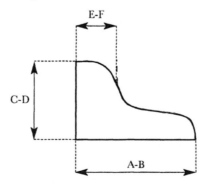

Figure 7.7 Design for a simple lateral support.

Weakness

Muscle weakness affects the control of the trunk and head whilst sitting; an individual can slump forward with the head on the chest or sideways. Supportive cushioning and postural support equipment are useful to people with this problem. A chair with the facility to tilt in space will negate some of the effect of gravity, but again not everybody feels able to interact with his/her environment adequately in a tilted position. Poor head control can result in the head falling into any position if no support is provided. If the correct head and lateral supports are set into the backrest of the wheelchair, the head can only fall forwards onto the chest. There are a variety of solutions to this but none of them is easy for the person to use. A cervical collar (any of the standard models) will hold the head erect, but these become hot and uncomfortable and some inhibit swallowing. Head restraints are available in a range of technical sophistication and cost, but are often rejected on cosmetic grounds. The most frequently used design involves a band worn round the forehead and fixed either to the headrest of the chair or to independent struts. Some people will accept a baseball cap worn back to front that can be fastened to the backrest of the wheelchair. However, the most effective solution is seating with tilt in space so that gravity can be excluded from the situation. Ideally a tilt in space chair should have electrically powered tilt so that the person has control of the angle of tilt.

Wind Sweep

Wind sweep is a descriptive term used for the deviation of both legs from the hips to one side in the wheelchair (see Figure 7.1). Usually this is due to inadequate support of the legs in early wheelchair use and can be associated with mild dementia. The person needs to be correctly positioned with supportive cushioning and reminded to maintain the corrected position. The help of family and carers may need to be enlisted to maintain the change of posture until it becomes familiar to the individual.

Adduction of Hips

Powerful spasm in the adductor muscles of the hips can cause the thighs to be tightly pressed together; it is common in the later stages of MS and presents a major hygiene problem. Action that will be of some assistance can be taken while the person is sitting in the wheelchair. A V-shaped wedge of foam is placed between the knees, in order to prevent the hips becoming fixed in the very tightly adducted position. The foam will need to be firm enough to resist the powerful adduction, but soft enough to avoid pressure problems. As with any piece of equipment that is added to the wheelchair, regular checks of pressure area integrity are essential.

Cervical Kyphosis

Cervical kyphosis is a fixed deformity of the neck; sometimes known as 'dowager's hump', it is brought about by prolonged lifting of the head, on a static trunk, to look above eye level. This can ultimately produce the symptoms of constriction of the spinal cord, and sometimes sensory problems of the hands that are hard to distinguish from similar symptoms directly due to MS. Some assistance can be provided by making a habit of sitting to converse with a vulnerable person and encouraging others to do so too. A home visit will help to ensure that facilities such as the television and computer are positioned at or below eye level.

Electrically Powered Wheelchairs

Electrically powered wheelchairs are manufactured in a wide variety of styles and prices. Those that are designed for indoor use have small wheels with smooth tyres that move easily on carpet, and their batteries generally have a limited range on one charge. Indoor/outdoor electric wheelchairs (the acronym EPIOC is used by the NHS wheelchair services) represent a compromise between accessibility about the home and being rugged enough for normal outdoor use. In the UK a limited number of these chairs have been available through the NHS since 1996. Access to them has been shown to give people independence and control of their occupations, allowing them to 'experience life, expand their roles and facilitate social participation' (Evans, 2000). Franks et al. (2000) found that 50% of EPIOC users undertook new activities, with shopping and visiting friends and family the most common. They also found that the majority of EPIOC users felt that the chair had helped carers by increasing their independence, and reducing pushing and transfers. Neither of these studies was specific to people with MS but a proportion of their samples would have been people with MS.

There are also electrically powered outdoor wheelchairs that can only be used outside because they are too big to gain useful access to the home. They often have a very long range on one charge of the batteries, tend to have more substantial seats and are therefore more comfortable than the dual-purpose wheelchair. One final option is the power-assisted wheelchair, a self-propelling wheelchair to which a motor and battery can be fitted. These have the advantage of being easy to transport and do not create any additional access problems. Power-assisted wheelchairs only use a 12-volt battery and have a limited range but can be useful for some people. They can provide some power to assist propulsion when the person with MS experiences fatigue, and can also help carers with hills and when they are tired. Propulsion can be achieved through the addition of a small control box and joystick or a link to the propelling wheels so that each push of the wheels produces a burst of power.

Any potential user of an electrically powered wheelchair should be measured in the same way as for an ordinary wheelchair, as discussed earlier in this chapter. He/she should also be assessed in an electric wheelchair; this should be done in a large open space where the individual will be able to practise once the controls have been explained. The user should then be asked to negotiate obstacles, drive through a doorway and up and down a ramp. A computer-based joystick game can be used to simulate the movement of driving an electric wheelchair, making practice in the occupational therapy department possible and fun. Not everybody with MS who is sufficiently disabled to need electrically powered mobility will have the perceptual skills to drive such a chair, and if there is any doubt a reassessment of perceptual function will be necessary. Visual problems can also make the person dangerous to him- or herself and to other people.

The vast majority of electric wheelchairs are powered by two 12-volt batteries connected in series, which need to be recharged at regular intervals depending on the distance that the individual travels in the chair. It is possible for this to vary from a few hundred yards about the house to several miles. With older electric wheelchairs it is recommended that the charging does not take place at night in the person's bedroom, as there is a possibility of toxic fumes being emitted during the charging process. This is a problem for some people who live alone and are dependent upon their electric wheelchair at all times. New chairs are fitted with gel batteries as standard; these are completely sealed, cause no fumes and can be charged anywhere.

The person who plans to buy her/his own electric wheelchair has a wide variety of choice, limited only by the individual's disability and finances. It will be necessary to make some choices and compromises, and these will depend on the user's desired lifestyle. The occupational therapist needs to know the types of powered chair available, and the services provided by local suppliers. The person can then be helped to prioritize the daily activities that would be enhanced by electric mobility, and then make his/her own choice.

When looking for the right wheelchair with a patient the occupational therapist should also consider the likelihood of the person losing manual dexterity to the point at which she/he cannot drive with a standard joystick. Other modes of control are available – for example chin control and pneumatic control – and if the person might reach this situation she/he should be encouraged to choose a chair that can be adapted for use with these controls. People should also be encouraged to consider whether they will want to transport their wheelchair or always use it straight from home. Some powered chairs can be disassembled for transport in the boot of an average-sized car. Other larger and usually more sophisticated models can only be transported in a specially adapted vehicle. Transport is now looked upon as a big issue. The Medical Devices Agency (2000) has taken over responsibility for its regulation and has drafted guidelines, and the specialist suppliers look upon these as legislative. The following points from the MDA publication may be relevant to people with MS and the occupational therapists who treat them:

- There is a need for improved communication between manufacturers, users and service providers.
- Transport of the wheelchair should be an issue in the initial and ongoing assessments.
- Where a wheelchair user can transfer to a vehicle seat he/she should do so.
- Wheelchair tie-down and occupant restraint systems vary and one type will not suit all vehicles. Where numbers of wheelchair users are transported in their wheelchairs sufficient and varied systems should be available.
- Accessories and unoccupied wheelchairs should be secured safely and not block gangways.
- Scooters should always be transported unoccupied.
- An approved repairer should check wheelchairs and scooters that have been involved in a vehicle impact whilst being transported, before they are used again.
- Travelling with a lap-strap as the only occupant restraint is not recommended.
- Methods of restraint and risk assessment are discussed but the MDA insists that the advice should not 'limit access to, and

availability of, motor transportation for wheelchair users'
(Medical Devices Agency, 2000, p. 12).

Suppliers of electric wheelchairs have a national association and a
code of practice that requires them to accept liability for the safety of
an individual in a wheelchair that they have sold. Details of this association will be found in Chapter 11.

Electrically Powered Scooters

The electrically powered scooter is a popular form of outdoor transport. The range can be up to 12 miles on one battery charge,
depending on the model and the terrain that it will be required to
work in. The scooter is controlled in a similar way to a bicycle, with
handlebars, and therefore usually requires less practice before use.
Experience has shown that the public perception of a person driving
a scooter is different from that of a person propelling a wheelchair.
The scooter driver tends to receive more communication and is less
stigmatized by society. The scooter, however, is not ideal for people
with MS once they begin to have severe problems with muscle tone.
Transfers to and from a scooter are more difficult than from a wheelchair; there is little scope for adaptation of the seats and virtually no
facility to modify the footplate. Both scooter and electric wheelchair
users could be liable for personal injury claims resulting from hitting
a member of the public while driving the vehicle. Whilst the person
is being assessed and helped to choose powered mobility, he/she
should be advised to obtain third-party insurance.

The Road Traffic Act 1988

The Road Traffic Act 1988 – The Use of Invalid Carriages on the
Highway: Regulations – applies to all wheelchairs. It divides them
into three categories:

*   Class 1. An invalid carriage that is not mechanically propelled,
    i.e. a manual wheelchair.
*   Class 2. A mechanically propelled invalid carriage that is not
    capable of speeds in excess of 4 mph.
*   Class 3. A mechanically propelled invalid carriage that is
    capable of speeds in excess of 4 mph but incapable of speeds
    above 8 mph.

Most regulations apply only to class 3 vehicles; these should not be driven by anyone under 14 years of age, and if driven on the pavement should not exceed 4 mph. The legislation requires a speed regulator and a speed indicator to be fitted to such vehicles. There are weight limits set for vehicles and requirements about the effectiveness of brakes and parking brakes. When using the road in the dark lights must be used. If a horn is fitted it must not be sounded when the user is stationary on the road unless the person is in danger, or in motion on the road between the hours of 23.30 p.m. and 07.00 a.m.

Wheelchair Cushions

In sitting, 75% of the body weight is distributed through the thighs and buttocks. The cushion is therefore a vital part of any wheelchair assessment, and should provide comfort, stability and pressure relief. The range of wheelchair cushions available to people with MS is constantly being changed and improved; many are stated to be rigorously tested and indicate the level of pressure care that they provide. However, there is currently no evidence of a scientific basis for these claims and there are no standards. All the evidence of effectiveness appears to be based on the comparison of cushions in practice. Work is currently being undertaken at University College, London to produce international cushion standards. This section will not discuss specific cushions but will consider the three most common components of cushions – air, gel and foam – and also some basic facts about their use.

Air Cushions

Air cushions, of which the best known and arguably most effective is ROHO, consist of an ergonomically shaped outer shell that is inflated with air using a pump. Air cushions, while excellent for pressure care, are not good for postural support and impede side transfers. A good air cushion, if correctly inflated, will allow the individual with a pressure sore to sit without doing any further tissue damage. The setting of the cushion, that is the amount of air in it, is crucial and needs to be checked regularly; each cushion will have its own instructions. Where possible the person him/herself should be taught and reminded to make these checks. Where this is not possible it will fall initially to the occupational therapist to check inflation levels, to teach care staff or family how this is done and emphasize the importance of correct inflation. There is currently a school of thought that once a pressure sore has healed the air cushion should be replaced with a more posturally supportive cushion that will allow the vulnerable pressure areas to develop greater tissue viability, rather than always being totally protected. This is an ongoing dialogue between experts.

Gel Cushions

Gel cushions are made from a variety of complex jelly-like fluids that are engineered to absorb pressure and to conform to body contours; they are continually changing and improving. They provide good postural support and some are cool to sit on but they are heavy. Weight may be a problem if the cushion needs to be moved frequently and the individual does not have regular assistance. In the hospital setting a regular role for the occupational therapist is to ensure that cushions are placed in the chairs in the correct orientation, and to ensure staff are trained not to store them on their sides because some gel may migrate to one side of the cushion and stay there. This information will also need to be conveyed to the person, their family and paid carers.

Foam Cushions

Foam used to be the poor relation of cushion fillers. It is relatively inexpensive, easily cut with an electric knife and widely used in occupational therapy departments to make temporary adjustments to positioning. It is still used for the basic range of cushions where pressure is not a problem. Foam is also used in conjunction with gel in some seating systems. Its most recent use is in 'foam carve', that is a cushion or a seat insert cut from a mould to match the individual's body contours. This gives support evenly over the whole seating surface and minimizes pressure risks.

Assessment for a Cushion

The factors that have to be considered when assessing somebody for a cushion are:

(1) pressure score on the Waterlow scale (1988) or a suitable similar scale;
(2) the need for a supportive sitting position;
(3) the preferred method of transfer;
(4) the individual's level of activity;
(5) continence – problems with continence mean that there is a need for a suitable protective cover and comfort should be

ensured for those with catheters, which can be very uncomfortable, especially for females, if the cushion is too firm;

(6) the required sitting height both for lateral stability and transfers.
(7) temperature sensitivity – the need for a cool seat;
(8) whether the person can cope with the weight of the cushion;
(9) whether the person and or their family can cope with the main-
     tenance of the cushion.

Cushion Shapes

It is helpful for the occupational therapist who does not have regular
involvement with the provision of wheelchairs and cushions to be
aware of the shapes of cushions other than the standard squares and
rectangles.

•   A wedged cushion slopes in one line from high at the front to
    low but still protective at the back. A slope from back to front is
    used for people who need help with rising from the chair, not for
    those with muscle spasms that need to be controlled.
•   A ramped cushion is wedged from the front but flattens out 5 cm
    (2") in front of the ischial tuberosities, still allowing sufficient
    depth at the back to provide pressure care.
•   Ring cushions are readily available but have no place in the
    seating of people with MS; they exacerbate poor posture and
    concentrate pressure rather than relieving it.

Cushion Covers

Cushion covers need to be loose fitting over the cushion; if they are
too tight they reduce the effectiveness of the cushion. In the hospital
setting it is often necessary to remove incontinence sheets and draw
sheets from cushions, which requires some tactful education of the
care staff. The newer type of cushion cover has the ability to breathe
but does not pass moisture through to the inside.

Driving

Driving Assessment

If a person with MS begins to have difficulty with driving she/he
should be advised to contact a specialized mobility centre, where
expert advice and assessment may be obtained (addresses of the
mobility centres in the UK can be found in Chapter 11). The most
frequent problems that people experience with driving are visual,

loss of manual dexterity, cognitive problems and fatigue, especially in a hot car. It is the responsibility of every driver to notify the Driver and Vehicle Licensing Centre (DVLC) at once of any medical condition that may affect his/her driving. Neither the driving assessor nor the occupational therapist has any power to prevent a person from driving. Only the patient's general practitioner (GP) can do this, though if a professional is very concerned she/he may contact either the GP or the vehicle licensing authority, which will conduct its own enquiry with the GP. There is also a national government body that will conduct driving assessments for disabled people and advise on vehicle adaptations; this is the Mobility Advice and Vehicle Information Service (MAVIS), part of the disability unit of the Ministry of Employment and Transport of the Regions. An individual can contact the service and ask for a specialized driving assessment, although the ministry's officers work closely with the mobility centres and contact through them is often more effective.

Access to the Vehicle

Getting in and out of a car is probably the most difficult system of transfers that a person with MS has to perform. While a standing transfer is possible, the door can be used as support with a helper holding it to prevent it closing on the person's legs or fingers. A firm strut running along the roof of the car, possibly a roof rack, can be helpful. Once the individual is seated with the feet still on the ground, a good range of hip and knee flexion is necessary to get the legs into the car. This is easier in a two-door car, whose doors are wider. The turn of the body may be facilitated with a fabric slide, but this must be removed once the person is in position, for safety reasons. Some people with MS can manage car transfers with a sliding board but this requires arm strength and not everybody can manage to use one. Some carers find that a sliding board helps them to pull the person across the gap from wheelchair to car seat, but this is not easy and requires two carers to do it safely. For those who can manage to slide, most consider that a banana-shaped board is best for car transfers.

There are more sophisticated items of equipment on the market to assist with car transfers. It is possible to get front car seats that revolve through 90° and 180° for ease of transfer but the person will still need good hip and knee flexion to get the legs into the car. Other seats that move out from the car as well as turning are available but again they need the person's legs to be flexible. The ultimate solution is the 'Autochair', a wheelchair that can be connected to a support in the car and swung round and down using the power from the chair. If used by the car driver this requires him/her to be confident and have access to support if problems arise.

Adaptation of Vehicles

Advice on the adaptation of vehicles is available from specialist mobility centres or direct from MAVIS. Patients should always be advised to consult a specialist centre rather than a local garage. Where Motability cars are involved, adaptations have to be carried out by a centre approved by the Motability scheme. The adaptations most often required are hand controls and extra-light steering. A lot of people also need hoists to lift their manual or electric wheelchairs into the car.

Summary

(1) Measurement for walking sticks and frames.
(2) The first wheelchair – how to make the choice and avoid problems.
(3) Measurement for a wheelchair – the measurements to take and rationale for these.
(4) Wheelchairs in permanent use – special seating and positioning.
(5) Adapting wheelchairs for people with MS – assessment and temporary solutions to problems of posture.
(6) Electrically powered wheelchairs – types and assessment.
(7) Electrically powered scooters.
(8) Wheelchair cushions – types and assessment.
(9) The Road Traffic 1988.
(10) Driving assessment.
(11) Access to a vehicle – techniques and equipment.
(12) Adapting a vehicle.

Chapter 8
Multiple Sclerosis and the Home

The Home

Traditionally occupational therapy has played a central role in assisting disabled people to function with maximum independence in their own environment. Occupational therapists who work with people who have MS have an established role in advising on the adaptation of the home. This requires the occupational therapist to be able to assess the settings in which the individual functions, and to facilitate his or her ability to carry out the desired activities.

Home is a far more complex concept than just the place where a person lives. Despres (1991, p. 96) described it as: 'not neutral, associated with self-expression, physical and psychological security and control, ownership and investment, social status, permanence, continuity and cultural meaning'. All of these aspects can be part of the assessment of the individual's home, and the weight that the person gives to each aspect will be different. Self-expression is seen in design and colour scheme and the image that the individual wants to be surrounded by and present to the world; this may very definitely not include visible evidence of disability. Security and control become more important to people because they fear the loss of both as a result of their disease. The need for control may be the biggest barrier to achieving housing adaptations that will enable the person and his/her family to cope, whatever level the disability reaches. Ownership and investment in housing is seen in the same proportion of people with MS as in the general population, at least at the time of diagnosis. The fear exists for some people that their social status and that of their family may be reduced, by both the financial problems of disability and its visible signs. Permanence in housing may become more important as other facets of life become less secure. Cultural diversity may be reduced for people with MS because it is primarily a disease of Caucasian people.

Occupational therapists have access to a vast amount of information about the home and the adaptations that can be made to it to facilitate people with disabilities. MS presents a range of problems that may cover the whole spectrum of needs, and makes the solutions complex and challenging. The majority of people with MS receive the diagnosis in early middle age; that is after they have decided on their preferred lifestyle and chosen whether to buy a home or rent from the public or private sector. It is therefore probable that most patients will have a home and possibly a mortgage. They may also have experience of doing work or having it done within the home and be able to organize this. It is unusual for a young fit person to consider a potential home in terms of access for someone disabled. Therefore, immediately after diagnosis the home is unlikely to be ideal, unless it is newly built, in which case it should have level access to the property and to a toilet.

As part of the denial process people with MS can make housing choices that they find quite logical but which to the occupational therapist appear to be unwise, such as insisting on a two-storey home because stair climbing helps to maintain mobility. Even when stairs are becoming difficult people may insist that they can manage one or two steps and ask for a stair lift that does not serve the whole flight. The occupational therapist must look at the person's home and environment with a view to the worst possible scenario. This will not be necessary for every person but there is no way to estimate the level of future disability for each individual. People may also act without the advice of an occupational therapist, and find themselves in a situation where they are in debt for an adaptation that is already unsuitable for them. An example of this problem is a woman who borrowed money to have a shower unit installed in her bathroom. Within one year she needed to use a wheelchair for all her mobility and could not access the shower tray from it.

Housing change may become necessary either because the existing home is not adaptable or for financial reasons. Although it is theoretically possible for income support to pay the interest on mortgages, it remains very difficult for people to cope financially as owner-occupiers on disability benefits. It may be necessary for people to make an application for rented social supported housing, and RADAR (see Chapter 11) produces a booklet entitled *Finding Appropriate Housing* that would be helpful to people in this position. The need for housing change may also be precipitated by marriage breakdown or by young adults with MS wishing to leave the family home. Moving home is not always an ideal solution because it can involve leaving established support networks and upheaval for the rest of the family, such as a change of school for any children.

Initial Advice about Housing

Advice on the choice of suitable housing should be part of the initial package of information that is made available to people with MS. MS Societies produce booklets and items on their websites that can be provided for people when necessary. Harmon (1997), *At Home with MS*, is particularly recommended, as she writes clearly and simply about lifestyle as well as housing. Unless their disease is rapidly progressive people will have psychological and emotional issues to work through before they come to be concerned about their housing, but it is vital that they know whom to contact when the need arises. Stress has been laid on those people who take an alternative view of their options to the established medical one, but most people will want unbiased information and advice to help them in decision making. The advice that is available can be summarized under the headings area, access, internal facilities and maintenance. People and their families can be advised to consider each point, its importance to them and its possible future relevance.

Area

People may have to decide on their priorities in terms of the area in which they live. Points that can be considered are:

- Beauty of surroundings tends to go with uneven terrain and distance from amenities.
- It may be important to live close to family and friends who can help in times of need.
- The availability of public transport may be important if the person does not drive – or may not always be able to. The availability of easy-access buses may become important.
- People may also want to consider whether they feel safe and secure in their home; city centres close to amenities are seen as less safe. People on their own or in the later stages of MS may

feel more secure in warden-controlled accommodation or an apartment block that has a video entry phone.

Access

- Level access to the home is ideal but not easy to find, except in newly built houses. If this cannot be achieved, those with MS should look for housing with a minimal number of steps that can be ramped easily, using the ratio of at least 1:20 for ease of self-propulsion.
- If the home is a flat in a high-rise block it is vital to the person's independence that the lift is known to be reliable, ideally with secure external doors and a telephone entry system.
- A garden should also be taken into consideration: first as to whether the person actually wants one, and if so whether it can be made accessible and be adapted for ease of maintenance.
- Outdoor storage space may be necessary for a scooter or outdoor wheelchair.
- For a driver it is important that parking space is available close to the property and that the terrain between the parking space and the house is free from steps and other hazards to walking or self-propelling a wheelchair.

Internal Features

Features to be considered in a potential home are:

- Good circulation space, with no internal steps between rooms and doors 900 mm wide to facilitate the propulsion of a wheelchair. This is particularly necessary in the bathroom, as circulation space will be especially important there.
- The possibility of adapting a ground-floor room into a bedroom if necessary should be considered.
- The stairs will be much easier to adapt if they consist of one straight flight.
- Walls should be suitable for the necessary fixings to put grab-rails in the appropriate places. This can include good quality dry lining but older more rural materials such as cob should be avoided.
- Heating is important to people with MS; those who are more severely disabled need a warm house because they are not able to move around and keep warm. Alternatively those with fatigue need a cooler temperature. Central heating is usually little more

expensive to run than a collection of assorted heating appli-
ances. In some countries but on rare occasions in the UK air
conditioning may be therapeutic, especially for people with
fatigue.
• Storage space is important to people with disability, who tend to
  have a lot of extra equipment to assist with the activities of daily
  living.

Maintenance

• It is important to consider how much maintenance a property
  will need from year to year, whether the family would be able to
  cope with this and if not, would this work be expensive.

Fire precautions

• It is also important for people with MS to consider fire precautions; it is more difficult for them to make a rapid escape from
  the house if a fire occurs. Smoke detectors need to be fitted and
  exit doors need to be easy to use in an emergency situation. Fire
  is a particular danger to people who cannot use stairs in an
  emergency, if they live in blocks of flats where the lift cannot be
  used during a fire.

The Background to Intervention

In the UK, help for people who need to adapt their homes comes
through Social Services occupational therapists who will be working
with the Housing Department of the Local Authority, which is
responsible for Disabled Facilities Grants. They may also be asked to
make assessments for Housing Association schemes, although
Housing Associations have the power to use private occupational
therapists. There is also the possibility of help from housing repair
grants and grants from voluntary agencies. It is essential to the therapeutic relationship that the person with MS understands the system
that is being used, and the relationship of the occupational therapist
to the provider of that system. It is equally important for occupational therapists to be certain whether their role is as representative
of the patient or agent of the provider, and where the borders of
these two roles merge.

People with MS will be eligible for consideration for Disabled Facilities Grants, which have a current maximum (2002) of £20 000 and are means tested. The person is expected to remain in the adapted home for at least five years, and the adaptations are expected to be effective for this length of time. There is no way to determine that this will be the case for somebody with MS, unless the adaptations are made to cope with the most severe disability possible. It is to the patient's advantage to ensure that all necessary work is considered in one application, and also to be sure that their finances are stable. If for example a partner is planning to give up work and become a full-time carer, this decision should be confirmed before the financial assessment is made. The Disabled Facilities Grant is not a rapid process; the time limit allowed for the Housing Department to present its decision is six months. This can be a problem following a severe relapse, when it will be necessary for changes to the home environment to be made quickly. However, the longer time frame should ensure that solutions can be considered fully and not put into effect unless they will serve all foreseeable needs.

Home repair assistance grants of up to £2000 may be helpful to people with MS for small works, but the recipients need to be in receipt of Income Support or other benefits and live in their own or privately rented accommodation. Housing Associations can make alterations to the house for a disabled tenant, though some prefer to re-house such individuals in more suitable accommodation. This may be helpful for some people but for others, neighbours and local services are important to both the person with MS and her/his carers, and more accessible housing may not compensate for what is lost.

Areas where Adaptations may be Necessary

This section will include only aspects of home adaptation that are relevant to people with MS.

Access Steps and Stairs

While they are able to walk safely, most people with MS will cope better with shallow steps and a handrail than with a ramp. Weakness of the arms is likely to be present once a wheelchair is needed; ramps therefore need to be as shallow as possible in the available space. Regardless of the problems that it may create, it is never appropriate to provide a stair lift that does not cover the whole flight of stairs.

Bathrooms

Grab-rails beside the bath and toilet will be adequate for most people in the early stages of MS, when standing transfers are more likely than sliding transfers. Mechanical bath aids will be suitable until the legs cannot be bent sufficiently to reach a position seated over the bath. These aids need to be stable and not rely on the person being able to perform a sliding transfer, although some people will be able to use the transfer boards designed for people who cannot lift themselves. These have a separate seat that runs smoothly in a channel, so that the person can easily be pushed along it into position. When getting into a normal bath becomes impossible, the most practical adaptation is the level-floor shower. This can be used standing, seated on a flap-down bench or in a self-propelling wheelchair. In all seated positions care is necessary to ensure that the bottom and perineum can be washed adequately, as continence problems are likely to be present. Not everybody is happy to give up a bath for a shower. Side- and front-entry baths are ideal until the point is reached when transfer becomes too difficult. A hoist – either mobile or ceiling track – can be used for bathing but the process tends to be a cumbersome, involving wet slings and being moved elsewhere to dry.

Kitchens

A person with MS who needs to work in the kitchen and uses a wheelchair will require the kitchen to be adapted for wheelchair use. That is, with workstations where the wheelchair can be driven under a working surface, and continuous working surfaces so that hot or heavy items can be slid rather than lifted. The person with MS may not continue to be the main or sole user of the kitchen, and it can be awkward and uncomfortable for a carer to use the wheelchair-height working surface while standing. It may be a more successful solution to partially adapt the kitchen, leaving separate working areas for use when sitting or when standing.

Living Areas

Living areas need to have wide doorways – minimum 900 mm – and plenty of circulation space. Most people will, at some time in the course of their disease, use stable furniture to aid mobility about the house, while they are able to do so. This technique is often not acceptable to professionals but it clearly happens, and it is therefore important to ensure that furniture is sufficiently stable and well positioned for safety. Floor coverings can be important: some carpets make walking or wheelchair propulsion difficult. A person who needs to be careful in walking but who manages safely should be advised to make every effort to try walking on a floor covering before purchasing it.

Track Hoists

Ceiling-track hoists take up less space in the home, they are less cumbersome and easier for carers to use. However, they do necessitate transfers taking place in a given area: the bedroom to bathroom track will not serve an armchair in the sitting room or cope with a fall other than in the bedroom and bathroom area. The decision between a fixed ceiling-track hoist and a mobile one needs to be taken in discussion with everybody involved with its use.

Low Vision

The adaptations that may help people with MS who have problems with low vision include measures to increase safety in the home and to improve the lighting. Internal steps, doors that are often left open, heated installations and any other hazards should be protected or clearly marked. People with low vision who are mobile will prefer to be in contact with the walls or furniture and obstacles that could impede this progress should be moved.

The Negotiation of Compromise

As has already been stressed, people with MS are all individuals and have different approaches to their disability; they also live in homes that are different. There is therefore no formula for one perfect housing adaptation. The ideal situation is for the person with MS and her/his family to discuss their needs and preferences with the occupational therapist and reach a mutually agreed decision that can be presented to an expert in the necessary finance and building work. Dudman (1995) describes the occupational therapist considering the expressed needs of the disabled person, those identified by the family and an objective view of the possible prognosis. She describes the final, informed decision as resulting from the occupational therapist's skill and exercise of professional responsibility.

Social Service Departments and Housing Departments may have established policies to deal with situations where there is a difficulty in reconciling the patient's expressed needs and the occupational therapist's experience of that individual's possible future needs. For example work will only be recommended if it can be shown to take into consideration a possible deterioration in the person's condition. While probably producing a more effective adaptation, these policies may make the therapeutic relationship very difficult, and the occupational therapist will need all possible professional skills including tact and patience.

Case Studies

This chapter will conclude with four case studies, to describe the problems of different situations and attitudes. These are four adult women, all at different stages of MS, the first able to walk with the occasional aid of a stick, the second with rapidly progressive disease, the third in a severe relapse and the fourth in the latter stages of the disease, all subject to fatigue.

Mary

Mary is a young mother who lives in a three-storey terraced house with her husband who has a back condition, her teenage son and her elderly mother. She has primary progressive disease diagnosed about 10 years ago. She walks safely (although her gait is not steady after exercise) but suffers badly from fatigue. She is able to run her home and care for her family, although this contributes to the fatigue. She is articulate and intelligent and has taken a lot of trouble to find out as much information as she can about MS. Because she had learnt about the uncertain nature of MS, Mary wanted to be prepared for the worst. Any change that was made to her home or garden was made accessible for a wheelchair. Her kitchen has been adapted for use when sitting or standing and her ground-floor cloakroom has a level-floor shower. She has raised funds to buy an electric outdoor wheelchair so that she can shop and walk the dog whenever she wants to, even when she is fatigued.

She sounds perfect: no problems for the occupational therapist to overcome in negotiating with her and assessing her needs, her adaptations would make anybody's life easier and are done is such a way that they do not look like 'disabled facilities' – but does she actually need all these things? A problem for the community occupational therapist was that Mary has friends with MS and other disabilities. Some of these people wanted the same provision, although they are not able to contribute financially as she did. Others felt that she has too much, and that all this will make her lazy or more vulnerable to the progress of the disease.

Carol

Carol was a young woman living with her partner who was having difficulties coping with the changes in herself and in their relationship, and with their five-year-old daughter. Carol had only had her diagnosis of MS for less than three years but she was reliant on a wheelchair, with her knees in fixed flexion so that transfers were very difficult. When their housing situation became evident, they were living in privately rented accommodation. It was not possible to adapt this home adequately for Carol to have access and to be cared for by her team of home care workers. After much discussion between the family and the local Housing Association an application was made for social supported housing. Carol and her family had a high priority for such housing, but the only suitable property that was available was a flat on the 11th floor of a block. Carol and her partner were very doubtful about this. Although the actual accommodation could be made suitable for her needs, with the addition of bathroom adaptations and the widening of one door, they were reluctant to move into an unknown area. They were encouraged to visit the property several times, including late in the afternoon when the local children could be seen playing in and around the block, and the housing officer arranged for them to meet a neighbour. Eventually they decided that they would feel safe in this block and that the move would make a vast difference to Carol's care. Fortunately their little girl, who had only spent two terms at school, made the transition to a new school quite happily, but this had been a concern to both Carol and her partner.

Susan

A further consideration is the situation where a severe relapse changes the home circumstances. Susan has relapsing–remitting disease and was still in denial about her MS. She went up stairs on hands and knees, sometimes going into extensor spasm. To get out of bed she pushed her pillow onto the floor, rolled over falling onto it and then crawled to her wheelchair, which her husband carried upstairs, or she crawled to the bathroom. Her only bathroom was upstairs; downstairs there was one sitting room and a big kitchen. Both Susan and her husband had chosen the house so that she had some obstacles to overcome and 'keep her going'. Following a severe relapse, her extensor tone made life very hazardous for her; she would slide down the stairs on her stomach and reaching the bathroom became impossible. Susan was given little choice but to remain, reluctantly, in a rehabilitation unit, because of the dangers implicit in her home life. After some weeks the reduction of her extensor spasm meant that she could go home, with frequent day care and supervision from Social Services. She and her husband then decided to move. They found a bungalow that was nearer to the amenities so she was able to go out easily, she now has more energy for social activities, and both she and her husband say that they are more relaxed.

Moira

The final consideration is a person with chronic progressive disease, in the unfortunate minority who do become severely disabled, who have had adaptations to their homes made during the course of their disability but only to the level of the current need. Moira lived in a converted barn that she and her husband spent many years working to make perfect. It had a sitting room and a dining kitchen down-stairs, the only bathroom and toilet upstairs and virtually no garden. Some 10 years earlier when stair climbing became difficult she had a stair lift installed, but it did not serve the first two treads of the stairs that turned at 90° to the rest of the flight. As time passed she lost her husband and gradually had more and more difficulty in transferring onto the stair lift. Finally she reached the point when she could not get onto it, even with expert help, and the transfer at the top of the stairs was assessed to be hazardous. The suggestion of a through-floor lift was put to her, but because of the strong feelings of pride and achievement that she had about the house, she refused this. The ultimate, unsatisfactory solution was to have a bed and a commode in a corner of the sitting room. She said that she was content with this situation because it had been her choice. Her occupational ther-apists felt that they had failed her and that an unfortunate decision had been made 10 years previously. However, no alternative would have been acceptable to her at that time.

Summary

(1) Home has different meanings for different people.
(2) Advice about housing that can be offered to people with MS includes the preferred area, access when mobility is limited, internal features, maintenance and safety.
(3) The available grants and other help for adapting a home are mentioned.

(4) Areas where adaptations are likely to be important are discussed.
(5) The occasional necessity to negotiate compromise is discussed.
(6) Four case studies are presented, to illustrate some approaches to adapting the home.

Chapter 9
Continuing Care

Not everybody who is diagnosed with MS will become substantially handicapped, but the majority of those who do will be in contact with an occupational therapist. The issues that relate to the latter stages of the disease will be addressed in this chapter. These are:

(1) moving and handling;
(2) the prevention of potential pressure problems and oedema;
(3) helping the individual, where possible, to teach her/his own carers;
(4) environmental control equipment;
(5) liaison with other services;
(6) respite and residential care.

Moving and Handling

Moving and handling are circumscribed by law in the Manual Handling Operations Regulations (HSE, 1992) and applied to the practice of occupational therapy (College of Occupational Therapists, 1995); the application of the law has been described by Mandelstam (2001a, 2001b). The College of Occupational Therapists recommends that occupational therapists working in relevant areas should take appropriate postgraduate instruction in manual handling and the law relating thereto. This is particularly important for occupational therapists working with people who have MS. They will need to be able to make risk assessments of people with MS whose transfers are becoming questionable. They will also need to be able, when necessary, to introduce mechanical assistance for lifting with sensitivity and expertise. They will also need to be able to teach manual handling to colleagues, relatives and paid carers.

People with MS should be facilitated to transfer between bed, chair, wheelchair, toilet and bath, independently for as long as possible. For some people intensive discussion about the positioning of handrails may be necessary. A few people will be able to perform a sliding sideways transfer using either a straight or a curved board (with talc sprinkled on if they are unclothed), but these are the minority who retain arm strength. At some point it may become necessary for the occupational therapist to discuss the need for further assistance with transfers. A risk assessment must be performed and documented, using the guidelines provided by the Hospital Trust, Social Service Department, other employers or the College of Occupational Therapists. It must take into consideration the safety of the person with MS, his/her family carers and paid helpers, as well as their views and wishes. The move to mechanical lifting can be difficult for the individual to accept, and the situation is confused by the double standard applied to the safety requirements for paid carers and the lack of support for family carers. Once an occupational therapist has assessed the moving and handling techniques needed for a person, all paid carers will be expected to use the prescribed and documented techniques. However, there are no sanctions to persuade the family to use a safe method of moving their loved one.

Two reasons given by family carers, particularly husbands and wives, for a reluctance to use mechanical lifting are that it takes longer to use a hoist and that it will change their relationship with their spouse. The latter can be addressed by discussing the change; a manually aided transfer involves close physical contact that could be called a 'cuddle'. Therefore the task is to put the 'cuddle' back into the transfer: it is still possible to maximize physical contact when using mechanical assistance. The way in which the positioning of the sling is performed and the closeness as the lifted person is guided down to the new position can be used to maintain this contact.

To address the idea that 'it takes longer' requires a sensitive training programme. In fact the statement is true: it does take longer to position a sling, move the machine into place, fix the sling to the hoist and make the transfer. However, it is safer for the health of the carer, and may be an essential requirement if paid carers are working in the home. It is also safer for the health of the patient once she/he is unable to transfer with manual assistance and if taught correctly should be more comfortable for her/him. The change of technique is not likely to be achieved in one session explaining the mechanism and the fitting of slings. The carer needs to practise, initially with a fit cooperative person who can make suggestions to increase the comfort of the process. The carer should also be lifted by an expert who inspires confidence, which will give them an appreciation of the sensation of being hoisted and where the potentially uncomfortable stages and potential sore points are. One other negative aspect of being hoisted described by some disabled people is lack of dignity. This can be overcome by careful positioning and concern for the individual's rights. It should be addressed at the very first practice and reinforced with all carers.

The actual choice of hoist may be predetermined by the relevant health trust, and if so the occupational therapist will not be able to select the exact model that will be most appropriate for the individual patient. However, a general observation is that people with MS do not cope well with the Standaid type of hoist that has knee blocks and one sling round the upper body. Spasm in the hips and knees and general weakness put a lot of pressure on the sling and also, if it is badly fitting, on the axilla. Where this type of hoist is suitable it is much easier for toilet use, because the dress can be adjusted much more easily. Some people may need to make the choice between the small mobile hoist and the fixed ceiling track. The portable hoist requires more strength from the carer to move it but is more flexible, it can be used anywhere within the home where there is sufficient space, and some models will lift the person into a car. The fixed-track hoist is less cumbersome, does not take up space in the home, is easier for carers to use but can only operate between fixed points. Some people who are routinely lifted by hoist will remain seated on their sling once they have been positioned in a chair. Great care needs to be exercised with this procedure as it can contribute to pressure problems, especially if creased or too tightly stretched over a protective cushion.

Prevention of Pressure Problems

Pressure problems become very important to people who are severely disabled by their MS, and are unable to change their sitting or lying position at will. The most common problem areas for which an occupational therapist is consulted are the sacrum and buttocks, as a result of prolonged sitting, the hips from positioning in bed and the heels either from bed or from pressure created by wheelchair footrests. Pressure sores, once they develop, are difficult to heal and can shorten the person's remaining life span. It is therefore important to maintain a vigilant approach with an individual who is considered to be at risk. Pressure care is essentially a nursing activity but the occupational therapist will need to be aware of the causes of pressure problems, the measurement of risk and have a basic understanding of the treatment of pressure sores.

Causes of Pressure Sores

There are three causes of pressure sores, all of which can be exacerbated by the presence of dampness from either incontinence or sweating:

- pressure;
- shearing;
- friction.

Pressure in any area, if it exceeds that of the capillaries, can cause them to become obstructed. The tissue that they supply therefore becomes deprived of blood and eventually ischaemic tissue dies (Waterlow, 1988). Research has shown that there need only be a period of one to two hours before unrelieved excess pressure results in pathological changes.

Shearing results from tissue rubbing over the underlying bones. This destroys the capillary circulation, and very serious deep pressure sores occur when the lymphatic vessels are also damaged. Shearing may happen when the person slips down in a chair or a bed or is dragged rather than lifted.

Friction is similar to shearing, and where the top layer of the skin is stripped this leads to superficial ulcers. This is most common in the presence of a spasm where frequent involuntary movement takes place. If the withdrawal reflex happens whilst the person is in bed, the knee is caused to flex and the heel to be dragged over the sheet, potentially causing a pressure sore on the heel.

Measurement of Pressure

The actual pressure that a person creates while seated can be recorded by pressure mapping, which requires equipment that is only available in specialist units and through the wheelchair service. Small pressure monitors that will measure an area of up to approximately 10 cm (4") are available. These do not give an adequate

picture of an individual's seating needs, but are useful for the identification of the cause of pressure problems in unusual areas. There are
several scales designed to measure a person's level of risk of developing pressure sores, the best known of which is the Waterlow Scale
(Waterlow, 1987). This scale uses facts about the individual including
age, sex, weight, level of mobility, medication, diagnosis and
appetite, to provide a numerical score that indicates his/her level of
risk of developing pressure problems. It is used preventively as an
indicator of the level of nursing care necessary while people are in
bed, and the type of cushion and mattress that they need.

Treatment of Pressure Sores

The treatment of pressure sores is an area of nursing expertise and
the actual dressings will vary depending on the latest research
findings. The occupational therapist needs some understanding of
this area of expertise to gain the maximum advantage from collaboration between the two professions. It is important to know that most
dressings produce a lot of exudates and therefore bulky pads are
fixed *in situ* over the actual dressing. These pads enlarge the area that
needs to be protected from pressure by the cushion that is
prescribed.

Occupational Therapy Intervention for People with Pressure Sores

The most familiar request for occupational therapy assistance for
people who have pressure problems is for advice on the provision of
pressure relief cushions. The research and technology involved with
these is moving so rapidly that any information about individual
cushions would become dated within a matter of months. However,
cushions are well advertised and advice is usually available from
wheelchair specialists; ultimately, the Posture and Mobility Group,
whose address can be found in Chapter 11, can offer expert advice.
The occupational therapist's role does not end with the prescription
of the appropriate cushion. In the home environment it will be
necessary to teach the use and care of the cushion and to make sure
that all carers are aware of this information. In the ward situation
care staff need to be shown how to use and care for each type of
cushion. Even when this is done it will be a very remarkable ward if
the occupational therapist never finds an over-inflated Roho cushion
or a gel cushion leaning on its side against a wall. One of the most
difficult concepts to impress upon care staff is that cushion covers
and bed sheets, if necessary at all, need to be laid loosely over

pressure-relieving equipment. Tight sheets, draw sheets and covers will form a hammock over the expensive pressure-relieving material and nullify its effect. The same is true of the clothing that the person is wearing: thick ridges of elastic in underwear, skirts pulled tightly under the bottom and fabrics with no stretch all increase the risk of pressure problems. Thick incontinence pads should never be used with pressure-relieving cushions.

Sore heels are often associated with a spastic withdrawal reflex, they are caused mostly in bed and nursing staff should be able to obtain protective pads to prevent this problem or to facilitate healing. The occupational therapist will need some expertise in the properties of pressure-relieving mattresses. This can usually be obtained from a nurse specialist in pressure care, who should become an ally. Information is also available from the local Disabled Living Centre or the Hamilton Index, for which the address may be found in Chapter 11. However, occasionally heels are made sore by the footrests of the wheelchair, where the knees are pulled into flexion pushing the heels hard against heel straps or the apron front. These problems need to be anticipated and adaptations to the footrests designed. One suggestion would be a sheepskin apron. Rarely an individual will present with a pressure problem that does not initially appear to have a practical cause; for example, along the outside of the thigh due to items stowed down the side of the chair; handbags can be hard; pipes and cigarette lighters can easily cause pressure. To discover the cause of this type of problem the small portable pressure gauge mentioned above can be used, installed over the site and set to bleep when pressure is applied.

Oedema

Oedema is the retention of fluid in the body; in MS it is usually seen in the feet, ankles and legs. It is mainly due to gravity and seen in people who have severe disability and spend a lot of time seated with their legs dependent. Compston et al. (1993) stated that it was not appropriate to treat this type of oedema with diuretics because these are intended to treat oedema due to heart failure. The use of diuretics may result in reduced potassium levels and also increase urinary output, which may already be a problem. The treatment therefore involves change of posture, which can be achieved by standing if possible, tilt in space seating or regular, but brief, periods of bed rest. Oedema can be reduced by massage provided that the skin is not too fragile; there may be a role for the occupational therapist to teach this to the family and carers.

Helping the Person to Teach Their Own Carers

Control of their care is very important to severely physically disabled people with MS, and many are quite capable of instructing their carers at each stage of the process of daily care. They do, however, prefer continuity of care so that it is not necessary to talk through the minutiae of each activity, every day. The occupational therapist can help people to regain this control and the self-esteem to require respect from their carers. The role of the occupational therapist is quite simply to ask the person how they like their personal activities of daily living performed, and not to initiate any stage of the process without direction from the individual. People can be guided into using the vocabulary that carers understand, without embarrassment; in fact they are usually better at this than the professionals. They can also be helped to appreciate the nature of the task that is set; for example when the task is heavy or unsafe for either carer or patient, the occupational therapist can say 'I cannot do what you want, in this way, on my own'. They can then discuss alternative methods and the possibility of additional help. This can be more acceptable from an occupational therapist, who is seen to be expert and has contacts with other caring agencies. This approach can carry over into the situation where the occupational therapist is asked to explain aspects of care to paid carers. The patient can be asked to lead the explanation, and the interaction between occupational therapist and patient can indicate the competence of the patient to control his or her care.

Environmental Control Equipment

Environmental control equipment is electronic hardware that performs functions around the home at the touch of a micro-switch. Information about environmental control equipment and service delivery for the UK and Europe can be found in the HEART report (de Witte et al., 1994). In most systems the patient has a control panel that indicates each of the functions performed and the status of that function. These control panels can be small and attached to the wheelchair or larger and freestanding in one or two rooms of the home. The patient will have a suitable micro-switch to activate the system. The basic functions of an environmental control system include emergency alarm, intercom between rooms and at the external doors, door opening, dialling and answering the telephone, switching on and controlling electrical equipment. In the UK, environmental control equipment is usually provided by the statutory services, that is the NHS or Social Services. Cowan and Turner-Smith (1999) found that these two services accounted for 75% of installations. Equipment is supplied to people who are severely handicapped, often those who live alone. It is expensive and requires an immediate response from the maintenance service; it is therefore too expensive for the average person with MS to install independently. For some small installations the local or national MS Society may help with funding but they will need to know why the statutory services are unable to provide the service.

Harmer and Bakheit (1999) conducted a small study of people with environmental control equipment, of whom nearly 70% had MS. This showed that the provision increased the independence of users and enhanced their feelings of self-worth and control of their environment; it also reduced the amount of care that they needed. They anticipated a rise in the number of systems provided in the future, because of the increase in the number of severely handicapped people living in the community since the Community Care Act (DHSS, 1990). Also they found evidence that health providers were becoming more sensitive to the needs of disabled people and their carers and quality of life issues. Technology is advancing rapidly, the range of functions that can be achieved by remote control is increasing, costs decreasing and the population, including people with MS, is becoming more computer literate.

The role of the occupational therapist will be only marginal to the actual provision of environmental control equipment, but she/he is likely to be involved in the initial suggestion that the patient is a suitable candidate for environmental control equipment and possibly the assessment for it. For this the occupational therapist needs an awareness of and familiarity with the equipment followed by assessment of the patient. It is important to be aware of the local protocol for requesting environmental control devices, and this information can be found from the local NHS Trust. It is also essential to know about the systems available and the amount of movement required in order to use each of the available microswitches. This information can be obtained initially from the Hamilton Index (see Chapter 11), which will give the names and addresses of suppliers who can provide further information. The equipment can be seen demonstrated at exhibitions such as

NAIDEX. This awareness comes before the assessment of the patient, because hopes and expectations should not be raised until the occupational therapist is confident that they have a practical chance of being realized.

The occupational therapist's assessment of the patient will have two aspects, first the determination of that person's most reliable residual movement and second the areas of need that could be met by environmental control equipment. The micro-switch required to operate environmental control equipment requires a small but positive movement that is reliable throughout the day. This can be almost any movement; examples are one finger, a knee, the tongue, or an eye blink. Most of these movements can be assessed with a simple micro-switch attached to a buzzer or a light bulb but specialist suppliers may be needed for the switches such as those controlled by eye blink that are more complex to set up and adjust. The movements required to activate the system need to be reliable over the course of the day, therefore the occupational therapist will need to assess several times, at least one of which should be bedtime. Here again, good relationships with the night nursing staff are invaluable. The results of this assessment need to be reported in writing to the person responsible for the provision of the equipment.

There will be a formal assessment by the approved suppliers. This involves a great many issues and people may find it difficult to follow and remember everything that is said to them and the questions asked of them. In order to make this process easier the occupational therapist can make the person aware of the facilities that are available from the equipment, discuss his/her needs and suggest that he/she makes notes of questions to ask the experts. One area that may be addressed is the person's reactions to stress, which could influence his/her need to have a learning period while the alarm is deactivated, as this is very loud, easy to activate accidentally and quite distressing if it proves difficult to turn off. Patients may also need to work through the idea of being able to let people into the home. In some areas of the country they will want to know that it is safe to open the outer doors by remote control.

Following the installation, micro-switches will have been positioned almost anywhere about the person's environment, with the aid of flexible poles, Velcro straps or more sophisticated engineered devices. Most people will require a switch attached to their wheelchair or beside their armchair and one beside the bed. The occupational therapist who has ongoing contact with the patient must ensure that carers are aware of the importance of precise positioning of these; if the person has difficulty in communicating, a small sketch can be attached to the equipment.

Liaison with Other Services

Occupational therapists who work regularly with people who have MS will find that there are many other services to liaise with when necessary. From within hospitals occupational therapists will need to liaise with several departments of Social Services, other specialist professionals and MS groups. Those who work for Social Services are often the first point of contact with the person who has MS. They are likely to have more information about the person's social situation and needs, but often find it difficult to make an in-depth assessment of the person's physical condition and skills in the personal activities of daily living. They may need to liaise with their colleagues in hospital to learn about any changes in the patient's condition and the need for further intervention.

In most cases Social Services will provide, or at least commission, home care services, adaptations to the home, respite and residential care. The needs of carers and particularly child carers have come to the fore in recent years. Social Services Departments are required to assess their needs as well those of the person with MS, and many provide support groups. These groups benefit from the inclusion of an occupational therapist in their structure. When dealing with home care, the occupational therapist is often in the position of being the only person involved in a liaison meeting who has actual practical experience of the individual's needs and the process of her/his care. Other agencies tend to be represented by managers or organizers who know what needs to be done but this does not come from personal experience. The occupational therapist will be able to provide accurate information about the patient's care needs and explain the importance of care techniques, such as stretching exercises, that are not a normal part of the home care services work. The occupational therapist may teach the appropriate techniques to home care workers either prior to discharge or during a home visit.

Specialist professionals include those involved with pressure care, continence and handling; the latter may be a physiotherapist or an occupational therapist, but the others will be nurses. There are also an increasing number of MS specialist nurses, attached to neurology and rehabilitation teams. With the pressure care specialist the occupational therapist will be able to exchange information about cushions, mattresses and positioning. The occupational therapy role in the maintenance of continence need only extend to the adaptation of clothing and positioning in the wheelchair to avoid pain from or pressure on a catheter tube. It is, however, useful to understand and be able to describe to new patients the services and equipment that can be provided. The handling instructor can be a valuable support in advising professional carers and in convincing a patient and his/her family that mechanical lifting will make their lives easier. The MS specialist nurse can be an ally with whom to discuss problems and evaluate solutions.

MS groups may require information and talks on specific topics that are of interest to their members. They are able to provide financial assistance with the purchase of equipment and possibly holidays. The occupational therapist may therefore be requested to produce a report in support of a request, and will of course have to obtain the person's permission before doing this. The occupational therapist who works regularly with people who have MS may feel the wish to help their local group with fund raising.

Residential and Respite Care

A small percentage of people with MS will eventually have to enter permanently a residential environment, which is likely to be either a client-centred establishment such as a Cheshire Foundation home, or a local nursing home that has registration to accept people under retirement age. Although the Care in the Community Act 1994 allows for greater resources to be made available for people with severe disabilities to receive care in their own homes, this is not always possible in the later stages of MS when admission to respite or residential care may be precipitated by a number of circumstances. These include the loss or illness of the carer, severe cognitive problems, increased medical needs such as deep pressure sores or percutaneous endoscopic gastrostomy (PEG) feeding. Also people's care needs may grow to exceed that which can be supplied, for example 24-hour supervision or lifting that, even with mechanical assistance, needs two or more carers. Any of these factors can be affected by the accessibility of the person's home, as regards both its internal layout and proximity to facilities.

Respite care describes admission to a care facility for a few days or weeks, mainly for the carer to take a break. The quality of care depends on the home that is used and it cannot be taken for granted that the patient will receive a medical and physical check during admission. The fear of ultimately having to enter a nursing home and lose control of their lives is very real to people becoming severely disabled by their MS. If people have already had periods of respite care they may have formed contacts within a home, which are said to make the move to permanent care more acceptable.

In the quarter of a century since residential care was described as 'a life apart' (Miller and Gwynne, 1972) too little has changed, except in a few areas of excellence. If admission does have to be considered, occupational therapists in health and social services should work together to consider all aspects of the person's social and care needs. Alternative strategies need to be considered, but once involved in the assessment and admission to residential care occupational therapists have a responsibility to ease the transition. Instruction may be necessary for nursing home staff if they are not experienced in the care of people with MS, particularly in handling and stretching exercises to facilitate personal care. It is also important to try to ensure that friends and MS Society contacts continue to visit and if possible arrange for outings and help to maintain contact with the outside world.

Summary

(1) The moving and handling of people with MS is discussed. The potential need to move to mechanical lifting and its accomplishment are considered.
(2) The causes of pressure problems are described and occupational therapy intervention in prevention and cure are discussed.
(3) The need to help people to teach their own carers is discussed.
(4) Environmental control systems and the occupational therapist's role in their prescription are described.
(5) Liaison with other services is discussed.
(6) The move to residential or respite care is discussed.

Chapter 10
Caring for People with Multiple Sclerosis

Just as no two people experience their MS in the same way, so their relatives, who may or may not need to become their carers, are individual in their attitudes to their loved one and MS. It is not possible to generalize about people's relationships but because they are frequently reported by people with MS and their carers, some problems can be accepted as likely to occur. This chapter will introduce some of the research work that has been undertaken into different aspects of relationships with a person with MS, and some of the things that people with MS have said about their relationships. These insights will not enable occupational therapists to say, 'I know how you are feeling'; however, they may prevent information given to them from being a surprise. They may enable occupational therapists to reflect back what has been said to them as part of a discussion and allow them to take some simple actions that could be helpful, such as referral to a carers' group. The problems of carers will be considered generally and the special circumstances that relate specifically to spouses and children will then be discussed.

The Caring Situation

Caring as a role in life has been the subject of much research. Twigg (1992) edited information on research into the numbers of carers and the practice of helping them. The statistics that are provided cannot easily be made specific to the carers of people with MS. One set of figures (Parker, 1992) that can be relevant is related to paid employment in the age group 46–65, the age group when MS is most likely to lead to severe disability, and when 64% of male carers and 54% of female carers are still in paid employment.

In the UK the interest aroused in the needs of carers culminated in The Carers (Recognition and Services) Act 1995, which gives legal recognition to the work that carers do. This entitles carers to request an assessment from Social Services when their cared-for person is assessed. The carer's needs must be taken into consideration when the Social Services Department is making decisions on the services to be provided for the disabled person. The Act is only applied fully in England and Wales; Scotland and Northern Ireland have other provisions. Wood and Watson (2000) describe the success of the Act as dependent on the ability of professional workers to find ways of meeting the needs identified in the carer's assessment. Their book *Working with Family Carers: A Guide to Good Practice*, is a valuable addition to the library of the occupational therapy department, and details can be found in Chapter 11.

Caring for People with Multiple Sclerosis

If people with MS become permanently disabled, it is often only the existence of a carer that enables them to remain at home. The literature tends to refer to the added tasks and difficulties that carers face, as a result of the caring role viewed as 'burdens' (Phillips et al., 1995). These burdens may be physical, psychological, emotional, social or financial. Carers are often left alone to provide a level of care that they have to learn about by experience and which would not be undertaken single-handedly by a trained professional. The burdens are generally seen as heavier for men than women. This is possibly because women have been traditionally seen in most cultures as the caregivers. Therefore the role carries social approbation, rather than the stigma that is often still felt to attach to a caring man.

Burnfield (1989b), writing for the MS Society, described some of the psychological symptoms that place increased stress on relationships. These include the grief, anger and depression that may result from the process of coming to accept MS. Relationships may also be strained by the fact of two people living very closely together with few emotional outlets. Cognitive problems can result in the person losing interest and confidence in meeting new people and undertaking new activities, thus also restricting the carer's social outlets. Problems with memory can be irritating and mean that the carer cannot rely on their relative for tasks such as relaying messages. In this situation the person with MS may also be offended, because she/he is not trusted with some responsibilities that she/he feels concern them or are important to them. This may result in conflict that in a few cases precipitates outbursts of anger, and possibly even violence, from either the carer or the person with MS.

The cognitive loss described by Lincoln (1981) portrays a person with MS who can converse and appear to be able and competent but who just cannot or does not perform the required activities. This presents different problems for carers: the inactivity of an apparently capable person can become frustrating and lead to arguments within the family. It may fall to the occupational therapist to explain this behaviour to the family, particularly because it is most likely to manifest itself in the area of activities of daily living. Burnfield (1989b) noted that once people realized that these problems were part of MS it became easier for them to cope.

Some carers remain in employment; they are likely to have fewer financial problems but much greater stress and worry about what is happening at home. Hospital appointments, medical and practical emergencies and the non-arrival of paid carers all need to be managed alongside the existing stress of the job. A person who is working and caring for a relative with MS needs to be valuable to an understanding employer. There are reported instances of carer burnout (Lindgren, 1990, p. 469), which occurs 'when a person fails to receive the expected reward or outcome from a job, way of life, or relationship'. It manifests itself in feelings of helplessness, uselessness and loneliness, an inability to complete tasks, loss of understanding for others and resentment towards the spouse. The factors that have been found to predict carer burnout are dependency in activities of daily living and household responsibility, and cognitive and behavioural disabilities (Zarit et al., 1986). This condition is seen more often in married partners than in other relationships and more often in women than in men.

Spouses of People with Multiple Sclerosis

For the spouse of someone with MS and progressive disease, greater demands will be made on them and their problems are likely to increase with the passage of time. The burdens of care seem to be greater for the caring husband than for the caring wife. O'Brien (1993) studied health-promoting behaviour in spouses giving care to people with MS. Health promotion was seen as a balanced diet, consulting a doctor about their own health, having any appropriate medical checks and taking stress-reduction measures. Wives were shown to take better care of their own health and to seek more support than husbands, who in addition to general support may need actual teaching on how to perform some tasks. Husbands were also assumed to be older, have been caring for longer and to be more likely to remain in employment.

Emotional effects of the diagnosis on the relationship can start very early in the course of the disease. One woman said, 'When they told us, my husband said that he felt as if he had already lost me'. A psychological state known as 'chronic sorrow' has been coined to describe the effects on the spouse of a person receiving a diagnosis such as MS that has an uncertain outcome and affects the whole lifestyle of the couple. Chronic sorrow (Hainsworth, 1996, p. 36) is defined as 'a pervasive sadness that is permanent, periodic and progressive in nature, it can result from the inability to mourn the fact of the disease'. Chronic illness requires a mourning process for the loss of abilities and lifetime potential, in order that the person can move on and adapt to his/her altered situation. Events such as anniversaries of the first symptoms or the actual diagnosis can exacerbate the carer's sorrow. Respondents to the study (Hainsworth (1996, p. 38) suggested coping strategies that included, 'trying to find humour in things', 'making an agreement with your spouse that feelings will always be open' and 'think of yourself, get out with other people'.

There are also the natural concerns of two people that MS will 'come between them' (Weiss, 1992) and inhibit their sexual relationship. Physical sexual dysfunction is a frequent symptom of MS, and one which couples find difficulty in ... ssing. It has been understood for many years ... ope better with the situation when t... heir difficulties (Barrett, 1976). Coup... ... to confide in whoever they feel it most comf... ... talk to. They should first be encouraged to talk to each other in a relaxed, stress-free atmosphere. A quiet evening in the local pub with a more experienced couple in a similar situation is probably the most helpful suggestion, prior to more private discussion. The MS Society produces a leaflet entitled *Relationships and Intimacy*, and a list of helpful books can be found in Chapter 11.

Children of a Parent with Multiple Sclerosis

The problems experienced by children with a parent who has MS can be both practical and emotional. These problems have been studied for many years; a classic paper was by Yuditsky and Kenyon (1979). Children and young people need nurturing input, example and guidance; if one parent is unwell it is possible that the other will be stressed and involved in his/her own emotional agenda. The child will then miss the important interaction of nurturing. The young person may have to do more household chores than are expected of his/her peers, to make up for what the unwell parent is unable to do. This may vary widely as the symptoms of the MS vary. Children may therefore have less free time and could miss out on learning how to structure their free time. They will have less time to spend with their friends, but friends will be very important to them. It is one of the strengths of children who have a parent with MS that they have the ability to make strong mature friendships and enjoy the company of their peers. This can become a particular problem for them if the family needs to move house in order to obtain accommodation suitable for the parent with MS.

Possibly because people do not want to upset children, but also because children have a talent for asking difficult questions, they tend to be excluded from discussions about the parent's illness. They are then unaware of the facts of MS, fearing the parent's deterioration and death or believing that MS is hereditary and fearing for their own future. It is natural that children in this situation will have negative feelings toward the parent with MS, who may not always be easy to live with. These feelings may also be directed towards the other parent and the family, and having these feelings may also give the child a sense of guilt. Blackford (1992) found that these problems and feelings could be helped by support from the well parent, a sibling or a grandparent.

Parents with MS tend to worry about the financial problems related to supplying their children with the things that they need for school and leisure. They are also concerned about not being well enough to support their children. Fatigue affects parental input: people can be too tired to attend school functions in the evening, fall asleep when they should be meeting the school bus, or be unable to sit on the beach because of the fatigue brought on by exposure to heat. 'You feel you are actually holding your family back, which causes stress because you can't do it. You feel guilty because you can't join in with them, then they feel they can't go and do something.' Crist (1992, p. 121) studied the interaction between mothers with MS and their daughters. Having reminded her readers that the treatment goals of occupational therapy 'should focus on lifelong living', she concluded that the occupational therapist can: 'promote healthy engagement in future parenting tasks by helping clients focus on treatment not only for the acute exacerbation period of the illness but also for lifelong adjustment in their parenting role (Crist, 1992, p. 129).

Children of people with MS need honest, simply written and explained information about the disease, its symptoms, the likelihood of severe disability and the slight probability of a hereditary link. The national MS societies now provide booklets of this nature; the one available in the UK is entitled *Has Your Mum or Dad got MS*. Children need to be included in family discussions and hospital visits, and they need to be aware of their parents' current problems. This may in fact help the 'fit' parent, who will no longer have 'to be brave' for the children. The second priority is for time and space to nurture their friendships, so that they have peer support. Blackford (1992) emphasized the importance of parents being aware and facilitating this need. She also recommended setting up a group for children of a similar age so that they could vent their feelings and gain health education. This would seem to be an area where occupational therapy involvement would be appropriate.

Summary

(1) The Carers (Recognition and Services) Act 1995 requires assessment for the carer when his/her cared-for person is assessed.
(2) The carers of people with MS face problems or 'burdens' that can be physical, psychological, emotional, social or financial.
(3) For a few carers these problems may result in violence or burnout.
(4) Spouses caring for people with MS also contend with the possibility of 'chronic sorrow' and worries about their sexual relationship.
(5) The children of parents with MS have an extra emotional burden and workload. They need to be able to seek support from their peers.

Chapter 11
Contact Addresses

International Society

International Federation of Multiple Sclerosis Societies
10 Hendon Street
London W1R 7LJ
Tel: 020 7734 9120
Fax: 020 7287 2587
Email: info@ifmss.org.uk
'World of MS' Website: http://www.ifmss.org.uk

National Multiple Sclerosis Societies

Australia

National MS Society of Australia
34 Jackson Lane
Victoria 3142
Australia
Tel: (613) 9828 7222
Fax: (613) 9826 9054
Email: public@mssociety.com.au

Canada

MS Society of Canada
Suite 1000 250 Bloor Street East
Toronto Ontario M4W 3P9
Canada
Tel: (1) 416 922 6065
Fax: (1) 416 922 7538
Email: info@mssociety.ca
http://www.mssoc.ca

France

Ligue Francais Contre la Sclérose en Plaques
40 rue Duranton
750 15 Paris
France
Tel: 1 53 98 98 80
Fax: 1 53 98 98 88
Email: info@ifsep.asso.fr
http://www.ifsep.asso.fr

Germany

Deutsche Multiple Sklerose Gesellschaft
Vahrenwalder Str. 205–207
30165 Hannover
Germany
Tel: 511 96 8340
Fax: 511 96 83450
Email: dmsg@social.de
http://www.dmsg.de

Great Britain and Northern Ireland

MS Society of Great Britain and Northern Ireland
The National Centre
372 Edgware Road
London NW2 6ND

National help line

Tel: 020 8438 0700
Fax: 020 8438 0701
Email: info@mssociety.org.uk
http://www.mssociety.org.uk

Scotland

Rural Centre
Ingliston
Edinburgh EH28 8NZ
Tel: 0131 472 4106
Fax: 0131 472 4099

Northern Ireland

The Resource Centre
34 Annadale Avenue
Belfast BT7 3JJ
Tel: 01232 802802
Fax: 01232 802803

Ireland

MS Society of Ireland
2 Sandymount Green
Dublin 4
Ireland
Tel: (353) 1 269 4599
Fax: (353) 1 269 3746
Email: mssoi@iol.ie
http://www.ms-society.ie

Israel

Israel MS Society
75 Yehuda Halevi Street
Tel Aviv 65796 Israel
Tel: (972) 3 560 9222
Fax: (972) 3 560 9224

The Netherlands

Multiple Sclerose Vereniging Netherland
Postbus 30470
2500 GL. Den Haag
The Netherlands
Tel: 70 374 77 77
Fax: 70 374 77 70

New Zealand

Multiple Sclerosis Society of New Zealand (Inc)
PO Box 2627
Wellington
New Zealand
Tel: (64) 4 499 4677
Fax: (64) 4 499 4675
Email: mssnz@clear.net.nz

Norway

Multipel Sklerose Forbundet 1 Norge
Sorkedalsveien 3
0369 Oslo
Norway
Tel: 22 604 960
Fax: 22 256 7695

South Africa

South African National MS Society
295 Villiers Road
Walmer
Port Elizabeth 6070
South Africa
Tel: (27) 41 581 2900
Fax: (27) 41 581 5705
Email: sanmss@jhb.lia.net

Sweden

NHR (Neurologiskt Handikappades Riksforbund)
PO Box 3284
S-103 65 Stockholm
Sweden
Tel: 8 677 70 10
Fax: 8 24 13 15

United States of America

National MS Society
733 Third Avenue
New York NY 10017
USA
Tel: (1) 212 986 3240
Fax: (1) 212 986 7981
Email: nat@nmss.org
http://www.nmss.org

Other Organizations Concerned with Multiple Sclerosis

Multiple Sclerosis Council for Clinical Practice Guidelines
Paralyzed Veterans of America
801 Eighteenth Street
NW Washington DC 20006-3517
USA

The MS Research Trust
Spirella Building Bridge Road
Letchworth
Herts SG6 4ET
UK
Tel: 01462 476700
Fax: 01462 476710

Advice and Information

The Disability Rights Handbook

Disability Alliance
First Floor East
Universal House
88–94 Wentworth Street
London E1 7SA
UK
Tel: 0207 247 8776

RADAR

RADAR
12 City Forum
250 City Road
London EC1V 8AF
UK
Tel: 0207 250 3222
Fax: 0207 250 0212
Email: radar@radar.org.uk
http://www.radar.org.uk

DIAL

Disability Information and Advice Line
Park Lodge
St Catherine's Hospital
Tickhill Road
South Yorkshire DN4 8QN
UK
Tel: 01302 310123
Fax: 01302 310404

REMAP

REMAP
'Hazeldene'
Ightham
Sevenoaks
Kent TN15 9AD
UK
Tel: 01732 883818

Disability Information Trust

The Disability Information Trust
Mary Marlborough Centre
Nuffield Orthopaedic Centre
Oxford OX3 7LD
UK
Tel: 01865 227592

Publication: *Equipment for Disabled People*

Disabled Living Foundation

The Disabled Living Foundation
380–384 Harrow Road
London W9 2HU
UK
Tel: 0207 289 6111

Publications: *The Hamilton Index*; books on dressing, gardening, kitchen, air travel

Specific Items of Equipment

T-Shaped positioning cushions
The Kirton Healthcare Group Ltd
23 Rookwood Way
Haverhill
Suffolk CB9 8PB
UK
Tel: 01440 705352
Fax: 01440 706199
Email: info@kirtonhealthcare.demon.co.uk
http://www.kirton-healthcare.co.uk

The Royal Hospital for Neuro-disability
West Hill
Putney
London SW15 3SW
UK
http://www.rhn.org.uk

The Neater Eater
Neater Solutions Ltd
13 Spencer Road
Buxton
Derbyshire SK17 9DX
UK
Tel: 01298 23882
http://www.neater.co.uk

Assessment Material

The Rivermead Behavioural Memory Test
The Thames Valley Test Company
Unit 22
Station Road
Thurston
Bury St Edmonds
Suffolk IP31 3QU
UK

Cognitive Assessment of Minnesota

Harcourt Publications Limited
Foots Cray High Street
Sidcup
Kent OA14 5HP
UK

Rivermead Perceptual Assessment Battery

NFER-Nelson
Darville House
2 Oxford Road East
Windsor
Berkshire SL4 1DF
UK

Chessington Occupational Therapy Neurological Assessment Battery (COTNAB)

Nottingham Rehab Supplies
Novara House
Excelsior Road
Ashby Park
Ashby de la Zouch
Leicestershire LE65 1NG
UK
Tel: 0845 120 4522
Fax: 01530 419 150
http://www.nrs-uk.co.uk

Therapeutic computer programs
Crick Software Ltd
35 Charter Gate
Quarry Park Close
Moulton Park
Northampton NN3 6QB
UK
Tel: 01604 671691
Fax: 01604 671692
Email: cgfl@cricksoft.com
http://www.clickergrids.com

Organizations that Provide Leisure Advice

Yoga

The Yoga for Health Foundation
Ickwell Bury
Biggleswade
Bedfordshire SG18 6EF
UK
Tel: 01767 627271

Riding

Riding for the Disabled
Lavinia Norfolk House
Avenue Road
NAC
Stoneleigh Park
Warwickshire CV8 2LY
UK
Tel: 024 76696501

Gardening

Thrive
The Geoffrey Udall Centre
Beech Hill
Reading RG7 2AT
UK
Tel: 0118 988 5688
Email: susant@thrive.org.uk
http://www.thrive.org.uk/

Horticulture Therapy
Chicago Botanic Gardens
1000 Lake Cook Road
Glencoe
IL 60022
USA
http://www.nsn.org/regio/cbglib/HorttherapyResources.html

American Horticultural Therapy Association
909 York Street
Denver
CO 80206
USA
Tel: (303) 331 3862

Canadian Horticultural Therapy Association
70 Westmount Road
Guelph
Ontario
N1H 5H8 Canada
Tel: (519) 822 9842

The National Trust
The addresses of local headquarters where access information is available can be obtained from the UK national centre:
The National Trust
36 Queen Anne's Gate
London SW1H 9AS
UK
Tel: 0207 222 9251
Fax: 0207 222 5097
Email: enquiries@ntrust.org.uk
http://www.nationaltrust.org.uk

NT Scotland
The National Trust Scotland
28 Charlotte Square
Edinburgh
Scotland

Countryside
The Countryside Commission
John Dower House
Crescent Place
Cheltenham
Gloucestershire GL50 3RA
UK
Tel: 01242 521381
Fax: 01242 584270

Publication: *Informal Countryside Recreation for Disabled People*

Sailing
Jubilee Sailing Trust
Hazel Road
Woolston
Southampton
Hampshire SO19 7GB
UK
Tel: 023 8044 9138
Fax: 023 8044 9145
Email: info@jst.org.uk
http://www.jst.org.uk

Sports Centres
The Sports Council
Information Centre
16 Upper Woburn Place
London WC1H 0QP
UK
Tel: 0207 388 1277
Fax: 0207 383 5740

Reading – Talking Books
The Listening Library
Room 50 12 Lant Street
London SE1
UK
Tel: 0207 407 9417

Organizations Involved with Wheelchairs

British Hospital Trades Association (BHTA)
1 Webbs Court
Buckhurst Avenue
Sevenoaks
Kent TN1 1LZ
UK
http://www.BHTA.com

The BHTA accredits individuals to assess for wheelchairs and has a code of practice for these accredited assessors. Note that it is individuals that are accredited not companies.

The Posture and Mobility Group
http://www.Posture-Mobility.FSNET.co.uk

The Medical Devices Agency
Wheeled Mobility Centre
241 Bristol Avenue
Bispham
Blackpool FY2 0BR
UK
Tel: 01253 596000
Fax: 01253 596177

Mobility Centres in the UK

Ministry of Transport

Mobility Advice and Vehicle Information Service (MAVIS)
Macadam Avenue Old Wokingham Road
Crowthorne
Berkshire RG45 6XD
UK
Tel: 01344 661000
Fax: 01344 661066

Banstead Mobility Centre
Damson Way Fountain Drive
Carshalton
Surrey SM5 4NR
UK
Tel: 0208 770 1151
Fax: 0208 770 1211

Birmingham Mobility Centre
Hillcrest Moseley Hall Hospital
Alcester Road
Birmingham B13 8JL
UK
Tel: 0121 442 3434
Fax: 0121 442 3435

Cornwall Friends Mobility Centre
Tehidy House
Royal Cornwall Hospital
Truro TR1 3LJ
UK
Tel: 01872 254920
Fax: 01872 254921

Derby Regional Mobility Centre
Kingsway Hospital
Kingsway
Derby DE22 3LZ
UK
Tel: 01332 371929
Fax: 01332 382377

Edinburgh Driving Assessment Service
Mobility Centre
Astley Ainslie Hospital
133 Grange Loan
Edinburgh EH9 2HL
Scotland
Tel: 0131 537 9192
Fax: 0131 537 9193

Kilverstone Mobility Assessment Centre
2 Napier Place Thetford
Norfolk IP24 3RL
UK
Tel: 01842 753029

Tyneside Mobility Centre
Regional Rehabilitation Centre
Hunters Road
Newcastle upon Tyne NE2 4NR
UK
Tel: 0191 219 5694
Fax: 0191 219 5665

Mobility Service of the Disabled Living Centre (West of England)
The Vassall Centre Gill Avenue
Fishponds
Bristol BS16 2QQ
UK
Tel: 0117 965 9353
Fax: 0117 965 3652

North Wales Disabled Drivers Assessment Centre
Glan Clwyd Hospital Bodelwyddan
Denbighshire LL18 5UJ
Wales
Tel: 01745 584858
Fax: 01745 582762

Northern Ireland Mobility Centre
Disability Action Transport Unit 1
22 Stockman's Way
Belfast BT9 7ET
Northern Ireland

Oxford Driving Assessment Centre
Mary Marlborough Centre
Windmill Road Headington
Oxford OX3 7LD
UK
Tel: 01865 227600
Fax: 01865 227294

South Wales Disabled Drivers Assessment Centre
Rookwood Hospital
Fairwater Road
Llandaff
Cardiff CF5 2YN
Wales
Tel: 029 2055 5130
Fax: 029 2055 5130

William Merritt Disabled Living Centre
St Mary's Hospital
Green Hill Road
Armley
Leeds LS12 3QE
UK
Tel: 0113 279 3140
Fax: 0113 231 9291

Wrightington Mobility Centre
Wrightington Hospital
Hall Lane
Appley Bridge
Wigan
Lancashire WN6 9EP
UK
Tel: 01257 256409
Fax: 01257 253809

Occupational Therapy Special Interest Groups

The UK special interest groups listed below all have interests that
are relevant to people with MS. Details of current contact numbers
for these groups can be found in the BAOT's *OT News*.

Clinical Interest Group in Orthotics Prosthetics and Wheelchairs
    (CIGOPW)
College of Occupational Therapists Special Section in Housing
    (COTSSIH)
National Association of Neurological Occupational Therapists
    (NANOT)
Occupational Therapy in Work Practice and Productivity (OTWPP)

Working with Carers

Publication: Wood J, Watson P. *Working with Family Carers: A Guide for
Professional Carers*
Age Concern
1268 London Road
London SW16 4ER
UK

Multiple Sclerosis and Sexuality

Sexual Problems of the Disabled (SPOD)
SPOD is the main source of help with sexual problems available to disabled people in the UK. It produces a wide variety of leaflets, some of them specific to MS and others that can also be useful. Counselling is also provided, either by telephone or in the person's home where practical. The national office will be able to identify the nearest local branch:
SPOD
286 Camden Road
London N7 0BJ
UK
Tel: 0207 607 8851

Publication: Barrett M. *Sexuality and Multiple Sclerosis*.
This booklet is available through the Canadian MS Society.

The MS societies produce leaflets and there are regular articles in *MS Matters*.

The following books are not written for people with MS but contain information and practical suggestions, some of which will be helpful to them:

Mooney TO, Cole TM, Chilgren RA (1976) *Sexual Options for Paraplegics and Quadriplegics*. Boston, MA: Little, Brown.
Rabin BJ (1980) *The Sensuous Wheeler. Sexual Adjustment for the Spinal Cord Injury*. San Francisco, CA: Multi Media Resource Centre.

References

Aisen ML, Arnold A, Baiges I, Maxwell S, Rosen M (1993) The effect of mechanical dampening loads on disabling action tremor. Neurology 43: 1346–50.

Aldersea P, Ham R, White E (1999) Wheelchair training needs for occupational therapists and physiotherapists. British Journal of Therapy and Rehabilitation 6(10): 510–615.

Anderson DW, Ellenberg JH, Leventhal CM (1992) Revised estimate of the prevalence of multiple sclerosis in the United States. Annals of Neurology 31: 333–6.

Archibald CJ, McGrath PJ, Ritvo PG, Fisk JD, Bhan V, Maxner CE, Murray TJ (1994) Pain prevalence severity and impact in a clinical sample of multiple sclerosis patients. Pain 58: 89–93.

Ashburn A, De Souza LH (1988) An approach to the management of multiple sclerosis. Physiotherapy Practice 4: 139–45.

Barer D, Edmans JA, Lincoln N (1990) Screening for perceptual problems in acute stroke patients. Clinical Rehabilitation 4: 1–11.

Barrett M (1976) Sexuality and Multiple Sclerosis. Toronto: National Multiple Sclerosis Society of Canada.

Beard JG, Ragheb MG (1980) Measuring leisure satisfaction. Journal of Leisure Research 12(1): 20–35.

Blackford KA (1992) Strategies for intervention and research with children or adolescents who have a parent with multiple sclerosis. AXON December: 50–4.

Bobath B (1985) Adult Hemiplegia: Evaluation and Treatment. London: Butterworth Heinemann Medical Books.

Bohannon RW, Smith MB (1987) Interrater reliability of a modified Ashworth Scale of muscle spasticity. Physical Therapy 67: 206–7.

Bowcher H, May M (1998) Occupational therapy for the management of fatigue in multiple sclerosis. British Journal of Occupational Therapy 61(11): 488–92.

Bracher M (2000) Theraputic horse riding: what has this to do with occupational therapists. British Journal of Occupational Therapy 63(6): 277–82.

Burnfield A (1989a) Multiple Sclerosis – the Case for Telling the Truth. London: MS Society of Great Britain and Northern Ireland [25 Effie Road, Fulham, London SW6 4HR].

Burnfield A (1989b) Psychological Symptoms and Relationships under Stress. London: MS Society of Great Britain and Northern Ireland.

Burnfield A (1989c) Coping with Fatigue in MS. London: MS Society of Great Britain and Northern Ireland.

Butler J (2000) Rehabilitation in severe ideomotor apraxia using sensory stimulation strategies: a single-case experimental design study. British Journal of Occupational Therapy 63(7): 319–32.

Coleman D, Iso-Ahola SE (1993) Leisure and health: the role of social support and self-determination. Journal of Leisure Research 25(2): 111–28.

College of Occupational Therapists (1995) Manual Handling Operations Regulations and their Application within Occupational Therapy. London: College of Occupational Therapists.

Compston AS, Langton Hewer R, Evans CD (1993) British Society of Rehabilitation Medicine: Multiple Sclerosis. A Working Party Report of the British Society of Rehabilitation Medicine. Oxford: Oxford Medical Publications.

Cookfair D, Fischer J, Rudick RA, and the MSCRG (1997) Fatigue severity in low disability MS patients participating in phase III trial of Avonex (INF-1a) for relapsing multiple sclerosis. Neurology 48(Suppl. 2): A173 (Abstract).

Cowan DA, Turner-Smith AR (1999) The user's perspective on the provision of electronic assistive technology: equipped for life. British Journal of Occupational Therapy 62(1): 2–6.

Crist P (1992) Contingent interaction during work and play tasks for mothers with multiple sclerosis and their daughters. American Journal of Occupational Therapy 47: 121–31.

Csikszentmihalyi M (1993) Activity and happiness: towards a science of occupation. Occupational Science 1(1): 38–42.

Cynkin S, Robinson AM (1990) Occupational Therapy and Activities Health: Towards Health Through Activities. Boston, MA: Little, Brown.

Davenport C (1922) Multiple sclerosis from the standpoint of geographic distribution and race. Archives of Neurology and Psychiatry 8: 51–8.

de Witte L, Knops H, Pyfers L, Roben R, Johnson I, Andrich R et al. (1994) European Service Delivery Systems in Rehabilitation Technology: HEART (Line C). Hoenbroek, The Netherlands: IRV.

Despres C (1991) The meaning of home: literature review and directions for future research and theoretical development. Journal of Architecture and Planning Research 8(2): 96–114.

DHSS (1990) Care in the Community Act. London: HMSO.

Di Bona L (2000) What are the benefits of leisure? An exploration using the leisure satisfaction scale. British Journal of Occupational Therapy 63(2): 50–8.

Di Fabio RP, Soderberg J, Choi T, Hansen CR, Schapiro RT (1998) Extended outpatient rehabilitation: its influence on symptom frequency, fatigue, and functional status for persons with progressive multiple sclerosis. Archives of Physical Medicine and Rehabilitation 79: 141–6.

Dick J (1984) Mini-mental state examination in neurological patients. Journal of Neurology, Neurosurgery and Psychiatry 47: 496–9.

Dresner J (1990) 'I can do that' or setting up and running a leisure activities course. British Journal of Occupational Therapy 53(5).

Drummond A (1990) Leisure activity after stroke. International Disability Studies 12: 157–60.

Duckworth S (2001) The empowerment approach. An extract from 'The Disabled

Person's Perspective', a speech given to a UNAM conference. Reported in the Newsletter of the OT in Work, Practice and Productivity Subgroup Summer: 7–8.

Dudman V (1995) Home assessment and housing adaptations. In Bumphrey EE (Ed) Community Practice. Englewood Cliffs, NJ: Prentice Hall, 116–83.

Dumazedier (1967) Quoted in: Parker S (1983) Leisure and Work. London: George Allen & Unwin.

Eachus P (1990) Health locus of control in student physiotherapists. Physiotherapy 76(1): 366–70.

Ebers GC (1994) Treatment of multiple sclerosis. Lancet 343: 275–9.

Elian M (1985) To tell or not to tell the diagnosis of multiple sclerosis. Lancet 6 July: 27–8.

Elian M (1987) Some aspects of stress in patients with multiple sclerosis. Stress Medicine 3: 263–5.

Esdaile SA, Madill HM (1993) Causal attributions: theoretical considerations and their relevance to occupational therapy practice and education. British Journal of Occupational Therapy 56(9): 330–4.

Evans R (2000) The effect of electrically powered indoor/outdoor wheelchairs on occupation: a study of users views. British Journal of Occupational Therapy 63(11): 547–53.

Evers KJ, Karnilowicz W (1996) Patient attitude as a function of disease state in multiple sclerosis. Social Science and Medicine 43(8): 1245–51.

Fairburn CG, Fairburn SM (1979) Relaxation training in psychiatric admission units. British Journal of Occupational Therapy November.

Finlayson M, Impey MW, Nicolle C, Edwards J (1998) Self-care, productivity and leisure limitations of people with multiple sclerosis in Manitoba. Canadian Journal of Occupational Therapy 65(5): 299–308.

Fisk JD, Pontefract A, Ritvo PG, Archibald CJ, Murray TJ (1994) The impact of fatigue on patients with multiple sclerosis. Canadian Journal of Neurological Science 21: 9–14.

Flanagan C (1994) Letts Guide to A Level Psychology. London: Letts Educational [Aldine House, Aldine Place, London W12 8AW].

Folstein MF, Folstein SE, McHugh PR (1975) 'Mini-Mental State': a practical method for grading the cognitive state of patients for the clinician. Journal of Psychiatric Research 12: 189–98.

Foster M (1996) Theoretical frameworks in the philosophy and history of occupational therapy. In Turner A, Foster M, Johnson HE (Eds) Occupational Therapy and Physical Dysfunction, 4th edn. Edinburgh: Churchill Livingstone.

Francis DA (1993) Current therapy of multiple sclerosis. Journal of Clinical Pharmacy and Therapeutics 18: 77–84.

Franklin GM, Burks JS (1985) Diagnosis and medical management of multiple sclerosis. In Maloney FP, Burks JS, Ringel SP (Eds) Interdisciplinary Rehabilitation of Multiple Sclerosis and Neuromuscular Disorders. Philadelphia, PA: JB Lippincott.

Franks AO, Ward J, Orwell NJ, McCullaugh C, Belcher M (2000) Introduction of a new NHS electric-powered indoor/outdoor wheelchair (EPIOC) service: risks and implications for prescribers. Clinical Rehabilitation 14: 665–73.

Freal JE, Kraft GH, Coryell JK (1984) Symptomatic fatigue in MS. Archives of Physical Medicine and Rehabilitation 65: 135–8.

Gibson BE (2000a) Stretching for People with MS. New York: National Multiple Sclerosis Society [733 Third Avenue, New York, NY 10017-3288].

Gibson BE (2000b) Stretching with a Helper for People with MS. New York: National Multiple Sclerosis Society.

Gilmore R, Strong J (1998) Pain and multiple sclerosis. British Journal of Occupational Therapy 61(4): 169–72.

Granger CV, Hamilton BB, Sherwin FS (1986) Guide for the Use of the Uniform Data Set for Medical Rehabilitation. Uniform Data Set for Medical Rehabilitation Project Office. Buffalo: Buffalo General Hospital, NY 14203, USA.

Grigsby J, Ayarbe SD, Kravcisin N, Busenbark D (1994) Working memory impairment among persons with chronic progressive multiple sclerosis. Journal of Neurology 241: 125–31.

Gulick EE (1989) Work performance of persons with multiple sclerosis: conditions that impede or enable the performance of work. International Journal of Nursing Studies 26(4): 301–11.

Gulick EE (1991) Reliability and validity of the work assessment scale for persons with multiple sclerosis. Nursing Research 40(2): 107–12.

Gulick EE (1992) Model for predicting work performance among persons with multiple sclerosis. Nursing Research 41(5): 266–72.

Haber A, LaRocca N (Eds) (1985) Minimal Record of Disability for Multiple Sclerosis. New York: National Multiple Sclerosis Society.

Hainsworth MA (1994) Living with multiple sclerosis: the experience of living with chronic sorrow. Journal of Neuroscience Nursing 26(4): 237–40.

Hainsworth MA (1996) Helping spouses with chronic sorrow relate to multiple sclerosis. Journal of Neuroscience Nursing 34(6): 36–40.

Ham R, Aldersea P, Porter D (1998) Wheelchair Users and Postural Seating. Edinburgh: Churchill Livingstone.

Handron DS (1993) Denial and serious chronic illness – a personal perspective. Perspectives in Psychiatric Care 29(1): 29–33.

Harmer J, Bakheit AMO (1999) The benefits of environmental control systems as perceived by disabled users and their carers. British Journal of Occupational Therapy 62(9): 394–8.

Harmon JE (1997) At Home with MS. New York: National MS Society.

Heller L, Keren O, Aloni R, Davidoff G (1992) An open trial of vacuum penile tumescence: constriction therapy for neurological impotence. Paraplegia 30: 550–3.

Hodges JR (1994) Cognitive Assessment for Clinicians. Oxford: Oxford Medical Publications.

Hommes OR (1997) Clinical and paraclinical diagnosis and classification: is staging of multiple sclerosis possible. In Abramsky O, Ovadia H (Eds) Frontiers in Multiple Sclerosis: Clinical Research and Therapy. London: Martin Dunitz.

HSE (1992) Manual Handling Operations Regulations. Sudbury, Suffolk: HSE Books [PO Box 1999, Sudbury CO10 6FS].

Hutter CDD, Laing P (1996) Multiple sclerosis: sunlight, diet, immunology and aetiology. Medical Hypotheses 46: 67–74.

Jablow MM (1998) Facts and Issues. Depression in MS. New York: National Multiple Sclerosis Society.

Jackson T (1991) An evaluation of the Mitchell method of simple relaxation for women with rheumatoid arthritis. British Journal of Occupational Therapy 54(3): 105–7.

Johnston M, Gilbert P, Partridge C, Collins J (1992) Changing perceived control in patients with physical disabilities: an intervention study with patients receiving rehabilitation. British Journal of Clinical Psychology 31: 89–94.

Katz S, Ford AB, Moskowitz RW, Jackson BA, Jaffe MW (1963) Studies of illness in
    the aged. The index of ADL: a standardised measure of biological and psy-
    chosocial function. Journal of the American Medical Association 185: 914–9.
Kaufman JE (1988) Leisure and anxiety: a study of retirees. Activities, Adaptation
    and Aging 11: 1–10.
Kidd D, Losseff NA, Thompson AJ (1995) The benefit of inpatient neurorehabilita-
    tion in multiple sclerosis. Clinical Rehabilitation 9: 198–203.
Kielhofner G (Ed) (1985) A Model of Human Occupation. Baltimore, MD:
    Williams & Wilkins.
Kielhofner G (1992) Conceptual Foundations of Occupational Therapy.
    Philadelphia, F.A. Davis.
Krupp L, Pollina DA (1996) Mechanisms and management of fatigue in progressive
    neurological disorders. Current Opinion in Neurology 9: 456–60.
Krupp L, Alvarez LA, LaRocca NG, Scheinberg LC (1988) Fatigue in multiple
    sclerosis. Archives of Neurology 45: 435–7.
Krupp L, La Rocca NG, Muil-Nash J, Scheinberg LC (1989) The Fatigue Severity
    Scale. Archives of Neurology 46: 1121–23.
Krupp L, Coyle PK, Doscher C, Miller A, Cross AH, Jandorf L, Halper J, Johnson
    B, Morgante L, Grimson R (1995) Fatigue in multiple sclerosis. Neurology 45:
    1956–61.
Kujala P, Portin R, Ruutiainen J (1996) Language functions in incipient decline in
    multiple sclerosis. Journal of the Neurological Sciences 141: 79–86.
Kurtzke JF (1955) A new scale for evaluating disability in multiple sclerosis.
    Neurology 5: 580–3.
Kurtzke JF (1983) Rating neurologic impairment in multiple sclerosis: an
    Expanded Disability Status Scale (EDSS). Neurology 33: 1444–52.
LaRocca NG, King M (2000) Solving cognitive problems: managing specific issues.
    New York: National Multiple Sclerosis Society.
Lechtenberg R (1988) Multiple Sclerosis Fact Book. Philadelphia, PA: F.A. Davis.
Lezak MD (1976) Neuropsychological Assessment. New York: Oxford University
    Press.
Liblau RS, Fontaine B (1998) Recent advances in immunology in MS. Current
    Opinion in Neurology 11(4): 293–8.
Lincoln N (1981) Discrepancies between capabilities and performance of activities
    of daily living in multiple sclerosis patients. International Rehabilitation
    Medicine 3: 84–8.
Lindgren CL (1990) Burnout and social support in family care-givers. West Journal
    of Nursing Research 12(4): 469–87.
Lubin FD, Reingold SC (1996) Defining the clinical course of multiple sclerosis.
    Neurology 46: 907–11.
Mahoney F, Bartel D (1965) Functional evaluation: the Bartel Index. Maryland
    State Medical Journal February: 61–5.
Mahoney P, Kannenberg K (1992) Writing functional goals. In Acquaviva JD (Ed)
    Effective Documentation for Occupational Therapy. Rockville, MD: American
    Occupational Therapy Association, 91–6.
Mandelstam M (2001a) Safe use of disability equipment and manual handling: legal
    aspects, Part 1: Disability equipment. British Journal of Occupational Therapy
    64(1): 9–16.
Mandelstam M (2001b) Safe use of disability equipment and manual handling: legal
    aspects, Part 2: Manual handling. British Journal of Occupational Therapy
    64(2): 73–80.

Mathiowetz V, Weber K, Kashman N, Volland G (1985) Adult norms for the nine-hole peg test of finger dexterity. Occupational Journal of Research 5: 24–37.

Matson RR, Brooks NA (1977) Adjusting to multiple sclerosis: an exploratory study. Social Science and Neurology 11: 245–50.

McDonald I (1995) Frontiers. MS Matters Issue 1(May/June) [MS Society, 25 Effie Street, London SW6 1EE].

McFadyen AK, Pratt J (1997) Understanding the statistical concept of measures of work performance. British Journal of Occupational Therapy 60(6): 279–84.

Medical Devices Agency (2000) Guidance on the safe transportation of wheelchair users seated in their wheelchairs. Blackpool: Wheeled Mobility Centre [241 Bristol Avenue, Bispham, Blackpool FY2 0BR].

Melzack R (1975) The McGill pain questionnaire: major properties and scoring methods. Pain 1: 277–99.

Mendez MF (1995) The neuropsychiatry of multiple sclerosis. Journal of Psychiatry in Medicine 25(2): 123–35.

Mertin J (1994) Rehabilitation in Multiple Sclerosis. Annals of Neurology 36: 130–3.

Miller EJ, Gwynne GV (1972) A Life Apart. London: Tavistock Publications.

Minden S (1994) Statistical profile. MS News 155: 12.

Ministry of Transport (1988) Road traffic: the use of invalid carriages on highway roads. London: HMSO.

Mitchell L (1977) Simple Relaxation: The Physiological Method for Easing Tension. London: John Murray.

Monks J (1989) Experiencing symptoms in chronic illness: fatigue in multiple sclerosis. International Disability Studies 11(2): 78–83.

Multiple Sclerosis Council for Clinical Practice Guidelines (1998) Fatigue in Multiple Sclerosis: Evidence Based Management Strategies for Fatigue in Multiple Sclerosis. Washington, DC: Paralyzed Veterans of America [801 Eighteenth Street, NW Washington, DC 20006-3517].

Multiple Sclerosis Society (1996) Notes for Professionals. London: MS Society of Great Britain and Northern Ireland [372 Edgware Road, London NW2 6ND].

Myers BJ (1995) Proprioceptive neuromuscular facilitation. In Trombly CA (Ed) Occupational Therapy for Physical Dysfunction. Baltimore, MD: Williams & Wilkins.

Neff WS (1985) Work and Human Behaviour, 3rd edn. New York: Aldine.

Neistadt ME (1992) Occupational therapy treatments for constructional deficits. American Journal of Occupational Therapy 46: 141–8.

O'Brien MT (1993) Multiple sclerosis: health-promoting behaviours of spousal caregivers. Journal of Neuroscience Nursing 25(2): 105–12.

O'Bryan GG (1972) The relationship between an individual's I–E orientation and information-seeking, learning and use of weight control relevant information. Dissertation Abstracts International 33(1-B): 447.

Parker G (1992) Carers: Research and Practice, Twigg J (Ed). London: HMSO.

Paschkes-Bell G, Da Cunha S, Hurry J (1996) Adapting to change when an employee becomes disabled. London: Royal National Institute for the Blind.

Petajan JH, Gappmaier E, White AT, Spencer MK, Mino L, Hicks RW (1996) Impact of aerobic training on fitness and quality of life in multiple sclerosis. Annals of Neurology 39(4): 432–41.

Phillips LR, Morrison B, Chase YM, Cromwell SL, Russell CK (1995) Effects of the situational context and interactional process on the quality of family care giving. Research in Nursing and Health 18: 205–16.

Porter B (1997) A review of intrathecal baclofen in the management of spasticity. British Journal of Nursing 6: 5.

Poser CM (1994) The epidemiology of multiple sclerosis: a general view. Annals of Neurology 36: 180–93.

Poser CM, Paty DW, Scheinberg L (1983) New diagnositc criteria for multiple sclerosis: guidelines for research proposals. Annals of Neurology 13: 227–31.

Prigadano GP, Fordyce DJ (1986) Cognitive dysfunction and psychological adjustment after brain injury. In Prigadano GP (Ed) Neuropsychological Rehabilitation after Brain Injury. Baltimore, MD: Johns Hopkins University Press, 1–17.

Quintana LA (1995) Evaluation of perception and cognition. In Trombly CA (Ed) Occupational Therapy for Physical Dysfunction. Baltimore, MD: Williams & Wilkins.

Rabin BJ (1980) The Sensuous Wheeler. Sexual Adjustment for the Spinal Cord Injury (SCI). San Francisco, CA: Multi Media Resource Center.

RADAR (2000) The Disability Discrimination Act 1995: Employment. London: Royal Association for Disability and Rehabilitation [12 City Forum, 250 City Road, London EC1V 8AF].

Reed K (1984) Models of Practice in Occupational Therapy. Baltimore, MD: Williams & Wilkins.

Reeves S (1995) Enjoy Good Food. London: Multiple Sclerosis Society.

Roberts MHW (1997) Multiple sclerosis. In Goodwill CJ, Chamberlain MA, Evans CD (Eds) Rehabilitation of the Physically Disabled Adult. Cheltenham: Stanley Thornes.

Rotter JB (1954) Social Learning and Clinical Psychology. Englewood Cliffs, NJ: Prentice Hall.

Rustad RA, DeGroot TL, Jungkutz ML, Freeberg KS, Borowick LG, Wanttie AM (1993) The Cognitive Assessment of Minnesota. Tucson, AZ: Therapy Skill Builders.

Sadovnick AD, Remick RA, Allen J, Swartz E, Yee IML, Eisen K, Farquhar R, Hashimoto SA, Hooge J, Kastrukoff LF, Morrison W, Nelson J, Oger J, Paty DW (1996) Depression and multiple sclerosis. Neurology 46: 628–32.

Schapiro RT, Baumhefner RW, Tourtellotte WW (1997) Multiple Sclerosis: A Clinical Viewpoint to Management. Multiple Sclerosis: Clinical and Pathogenic Basis. London: Chapman & Hall.

Schapiro RT, Langer SL (1994) Symptomatic therapy of multiple sclerosis. Current Opinion in Neurology 7: 229–33.

Scheinberg LC (1980) The employment status of 257 MS patients. New York State Journal of Medicine 80: 1395.

Scheinberg LC (1994) Therapeutic strategies. Annals of Neurology 36: 122.

Schwartz CE, Coulthard-Morris L, Qi Zeng (1996) Psychosocial correlates of fatigue in multiple sclerosis. Archives of Physical Medicine Rehabilitation 77: 165–70.

Shah S (1998) Modified Bartel Index. In Salek S (Ed) Compendium of Quality of Life Instruments. Boston, MA: Wiley.

Shah S, Muncer S, Griffin J, Elliott L (2000) The utility of the modified Bartel Index for traumatic brain injury rehabilitation and prognosis. British Journal of Occupational Therapy 63(10): 469–75.

Shah S, Vanclay F, Cooper B (1989) Prediciting discharge status at the commencement of stroke rehabilitation. Stroke 20: 766–9.

Siegel ME (1996) Hiring Help at Home. New York: National Multiple Sclerosis Society [733 Third Avenue, New York, NY 10017].

Silcox LI (2000) Fatigue in multiple sclerosis: the measurement of its management. Unpublished dissertation, University of Exeter, UK.

Siosteen A, Lundqvist C, Blomstrand C, Sullivan L, Sullivan M (1990) Sexual ability, activity, attitudes and satisfaction as part of adjustment to spinal-cord injured subjects. Paraplegia (Scotland) 28(5): 285–95.

Smits RCF, Emmen HH, Bertelsmann FW, Kulig BM, van Loene AC, Polman CH (1994) The effects of 4-aminopyridine on cognitive function in patients with multiple sclerosis. Neurology 44: 1701–5.

Sohlberg M, Mateer C (1989) Introduction to Cognitive Rehabilitation: Theory and Practice. New York: Guilford Press.

Staples D, Lincoln N (1979) Intellectual impairment in multiple sclerosis: and its relation to functional abilities. Rheumatology and Rehabilitation 18: 153–60.

Sullivan MJL, Dehoux E, Buchanan DC (1989) An approach to cognitive rehabilitation in multiple sclerosis. Canadian Journal of Rehabilitation 3(2): 77–85.

Thomas D, Daily B (1989) Neurology – What Shall I Do? London: Butterworth.

Thompson AJ (1996) Multiple sclerosis: symptomatic treatment. Journal of Neurology 243(8): 559–65.

Thurgood J (1999) The employment implications of the Disability Discrimination Act 1995 and a suggested format for developing reasonable adjustments. British Journal of Occupational Therapy 62(7): 290–4.

Trombly CA (1995) Occupational Therapy for Physical Dysfunction. Baltimore, MD: Williams & Wilkins.

Twigg J (1992) Carers: Research and Practice. London: HMSO.

Valleroy ML, Kraft GH (1984) Sexual dysfunction in MS. Archives of Physical Medicine and Rehabilitation 65: 125.

Vercoulen J, Hommes O, Swanink M, Jongen P, Fennis J, Galama J, van der Meer J, Bleijenberg G (1996) The measurement of fatigue in patients with multiple sclerosis. Archives of Neurology 53: 642–9.

Wade DT (1992) Measurement in Neurological Rehabilitation. Oxford: Oxford Medical Publications/Oxford University Press.

Walker VS (1987) Pain assessment charts in the management of chronic cancer pain. Palliative Medicine 1: 111–16.

Wallston BS, Wallston KA, Kaplan GD, Maides SA (1976) Development and validation of the health locus of control (HLC) scale. Journal of Consulting and Clinical Psychology 44(4): 580–5.

Walsh P, Walsh A (1987) Self-esteem and disease adpatation among multiple sclerosis patients. Journal of Social Psychology 127: 669.

Wantanbe Y, Bakheit AMO, McLellan DL (1998) A study of the effectiveness of botulinum toxin Type A (Dysport) in the management of muscle spasticity. Disability and Rehabilitation 20(2): 62–5.

Wassem R (1992) Self-efficacy as a predictor of adjustment to multiple sclerosis. Journal of Neuroscience Nursing 24(4): 224–9.

Waterlow J (1987) Calculating the risk. Nursing Times 83(39) 58–60.

Waterlow J (1988) Prevention is cheaper than cure. Nursing Times 84(25) 69–70.

Weinshenker B.G (1994) Natural history of multiple sclerosis. Annals of Neurology 36: 6–11.

Weiss J (1992) Multiple sclerosis: will it come between us? Sexual concerns of clients and their partners. Journal of Neuroscience Nursing 24(4): 190–3.

Welham L (1995) Occupational therapy for fatigue in patients with MS. British Journal of Occupational Therapy 58(12): 507–9.

Wilson BA, Cockburn J, Baddeley AD (1985) The Rivermead Behavioural Memory Test. Titchfield, Hants: Thames Valley Test Company.

Wilson BA, Cockburn J, Baddeley AD, Hierens RW (1989) The development and validation of a test battery for detecting and monitoring everyday memory problems. Journal of Clinical Experimental Neuropsychology 11: 855–70.

Wood C (1993) Mood change and perceptions of vitality: a comparison of the effects of relaxation, visualization and yoga. Journal of the Royal Society of Medicine 86: 254–8.

Wood J, Watson P (2000) Working with Family Carers: A Guide to Good Practice. London: Age Concern [1268 London Road, London SW16 4ER].

Yuditsky S, Kenyon G (1979) Family needs study for the MS society. In Opinions. North York, Ontario: York University Press.

Zarit SH, Todd PA, Zarit JM (1986) Subjective burden of husbands and wives as care-givers: a longitudinal study. Gerontologist 26(3): 260–6.

Zoltan B, Siev E, Freishtat B (1986) The Adult Stroke Patient: A Manual for Evaluation and Treatment of Perceptual and Cognitive Dysfunction. Thorofare, NJ: Slack.

Index

Printed in the United States
49468LVS00003B/277